Sexual Crime

Sexual Crime is an edited book series devised by a team at SOCAMRU led by Professor Belinda Winder in the Psychology Division at Nottingham Trent University.

It offers original contributions to specific avenues of research within the field of sexual crime with each volume drawing together a review of the literature from across disciplines, including cutting edge research and practice, original material from services and offenders themselves as well as future directions for research and practice.

These volumes will be highly relevant to clinical and forensic psychologists and therapists, offender managers and supervisors, social workers and those working in the field of rehabilitation. They will be a great source of insight for academics, researchers and students in these disciplines as well as criminologists and policy makers.

More information about this series at
http://www.palgrave.com/gp/series/15477

Helen Elliott • Kerensa Hocken
Rebecca Lievesley
Nicholas Blagden • Belinda Winder
Phil Banyard
Editors

Sexual Crime and Circles of Support and Accountability

palgrave
macmillan

Editors
Helen Elliott
Bishop Grosseteste University
Lincoln, UK

Kerensa Hocken
HMPPS Whatton
Whatton, UK

Rebecca Lievesley
Nottingham Trent University
Nottingham, UK

Nicholas Blagden
Nottingham Trent University
Nottingham, UK

Belinda Winder
Nottingham Trent University
Nottingham, UK

Phil Banyard
Nottingham Trent University
Nottingham, UK

Sexual Crime
ISBN 978-3-030-09083-8 ISBN 978-3-319-74823-8 (eBook)
https://doi.org/10.1007/978-3-319-74823-8

Cover illustration: Ruth Black/ Alamy Stock Photo

Printed on acid-free paper

This Palgrave Macmillan imprint is published by the registered company Springer International Publishing AG part of Springer Nature.
The registered company address is: Gewerbestrasse 11, 6330 Cham, Switzerland

Foreword

This book offers a welcome contribution to the literature and evidence base that is available on Circles of Support and Accountability (CoSA). The authors offer a fresh and interesting look at CoSA through offering perspectives on current literature and both published and unpublished research in the field. The book is relevant not just to psychologists, criminologists, social workers, Probation Officers and students, but to practitioners and the general public with an interest in learning how CoSA operates. It highlights the successful contribution CoSA makes to the rehabilitation of those who have committed sexual crime and those who engage in sexually harmful behaviour.

The publication of the book is timely as there has been a continuous grappling with the issues of how best to address sexual abuse in society, both in the UK and internationally. The statistics for sexual abuse continue to be disturbing. According to a study conducted by the Office for National Statistics there were 47,008 sexual offences reported against children between April 2014 and March 2015. In 2015, 8595 defendants were prosecuted for child sexual abuse, up from 7536 in 2014, a rise of 14%. There are approximately 49,466 registered sex offenders recorded as living in the UK as of March 2016[1] and an average of 3000 are released from prison every year.

It is important that we recognise that although it is crucial for us to continue to give help and support to victims of sexual abuse, we should also address the root causes of this behaviour, if we are to prevent further victims of sexual abuse and the devastating pain and trauma that this is continuing to create in societies and communities all over the world. We can only do this by working with those who have committed these crimes, through treatment and support programmes, of which CoSA are a recognised and respected intervention. It is this recognition that has enabled CoSA to expand significantly over the last few years and the initiative is now fully operational in Canada, the US, the UK, Ireland and a number of countries in Europe. In the UK alone there are now 16 Providers of CoSA, which are overseen by Circles UK as the national overarching organisation. We have also managed to establish CoSA in areas where they have not been delivered before, with the help of a Big Lottery funded project—this will enable the roll out of 188 additional CoSAs over the next two years—100 new in London alone. Our network of trusted and valued volunteers has continued to grow and we now have more than 500 active volunteers who deliver CoSA throughout England and Wales. These are significant achievements, and the publication of this book will add to our knowledge base and further inform the current debates and discourse on what is effective in reducing sexual reoffending.

The book is made up of eight diverse and highly relevant chapters. It starts with a summary of the historical development of CoSA, from its early beginnings in Canada, to the successful implementation in both the United Kingdom and Europe. This first chapter explores how the original model was adapted to a British context to ensure it became a meaningful component of the risk management process and highlights how this restorative community based initiative works effectively within the existing criminal justice system. Chapter 2 focuses on what we know about sexual offending and desistence from sexual crime. It specifically highlights the role of narrative identity in desistance from sexual deviance and how CoSA maps onto this. Chapter 3 addresses the issue that despite a growing body of research on the effectiveness of CoSA, particularly from Canada, the US, UK and the Netherlands, there is not yet enough evidence to determine whether they significantly reduce sexual recidivism. The author includes an overview of the key CoSA effectiveness studies carried out to date, along with an overview of future directions for research. Chapter 4 outlines the first prison-model of CoSA, which was established in the UK in 2014 and discusses some of the key findings from the evaluation. The chapter emphasises the importance of the support offered immediately on release from prison and the continued barriers individuals convicted of sexual crime face to successful reintegration into the community. Chapter 5 discusses the importance of evaluation and proposes a structure and process suitable for an evaluation of CoSA. Chapter 6 provides a fascinating overview of how the media shape societal attitudes towards sexual offending and makes suggestions to promote more constructive responses and debates that could help to more successfully address these complex issues. Chapter 7 gives a very personal insight into the thoughts, feelings and impressions of those most closely involved, namely CoSA Core Members and Volunteers. The final chapter of the book concludes with an exciting view of how CoSA may evolve and adapt in future. The authors focus on psychologically informed CoSA, specifically the attachment needs of individuals convicted of sexual crime and CoSA for non-offending individuals in the community who are concerned about their sexual thoughts or behaviour. The chapter also explores the concept and practicalities of CoSA for certain minority groups, including CoSA for transgender populations, deaf individuals and young people.

CEO Circles, UK Riana Taylor

Notes

1. Office for National Statistics: file://circlessbs/RedirectedFolders/EmmaB/Desktop/Focus%20on%20Violent%20Crime%20and%20Sexual%20Offences%20%20Year%20ending%20March%202015.pdf

Preface

This Series: Sexual Crime

This book series will offer original contributions to current books available on this fast growing area of high public interest. Each volume will comprehensively engage with current literature, and make efforts to access unpublished literature and data by key authors in the field. The series will also, by the end of each volume, suggest potential new directions for researchers and practitioners.

These volumes are relevant not just to psychologists, criminologists, social workers, final year undergraduate, postgraduate, doctoral students of all these areas, but to practitioners and the general public with an interest in learning more about the topic. The aim is to create books that are readable, yet firmly anchored in a sound evidence base from both researchers and practitioners. The volumes will include therefore a robust synthesis of the literature, consideration of the theories relevant to each topic, a focus on projects that are relevant to the topic, with a summary of the research and evaluation of these, chapters focusing on the service user voice and a final summary chapter, highlighting future possibilities and directions (as suggested by others in the field or by the authors themselves).

This Volume: Circles of Support and Accountability

The current volume offers a contribution to the growing interest and evidence base for Circles of Support and Accountability (CoSA). The volume highlights the theoretical underpinnings surrounding CoSA and how it contributes to the rehabilitation of those who have committed sexual crime and offers an overview of the literature to date. The book also provides original and unpublished research on CoSA, as well as a unique opportunity to hear about both the service user, volunteer and coordinators perspectives when engaging in CoSA. The perceptions of the public and influence of the media are also explored, and finally interesting and practical suggestions are made for the future of CoSA.

Future Texts

This series is ongoing, with planned future volumes including: sexual offender experience of imprisonment, the prevention of sexual crime and experiences of individuals living in the community with a sexual interest, spirituality and sexual crime, internet offending, sexual crime and personality disorder and the protective factors of sexual crime.

Lincoln, UK
Whatton, UK
Nottingham, UK

Helen Elliott
Kerensa Hocken
Rebecca Lievesley
Nicholas Blagden
Belinda Winder
Phil Banyard

Contents

1 **A History of the Development of Circles of Support and Accountability** 1
Chris Wilson

2 **Circles of Support and Accountability, Assisted Desistance and Community Transition** 25
Nicholas Blagden, Helen Elliott, and Rebecca Lievesley

3 **Do Circles of Support and Accountability Work? A Review of the Literature** 43
Rosie Kitson-Boyce

4 **The Prison-Based Model of Circles of Support and Accountability and its Application in Transitioning to the Community** 71
Rosie Kitson-Boyce

5 **Evaluating Community-Based Circles of Support and Accountability** 105
Michelle Dwerryhouse

6 **The Role of the Media in Shaping Responses to Sexual Offending** 127
Craig A. Harper

7 **A Different Life: The Experiences of Core Members and Volunteers on the Safer Living Foundations Circles of Support and Accountability** 151
Dave Potter

8 **Future Directions: Alternative Circles of Support and Accountability Models and Minority Groups** 171
Kerensa Hocken, Claire Good, Helen Elliott, Carrie Webb, Helen O'Connor, and Kim Cox

Glossary 201

Index 203

Notes on Contributors

Dr Nicholas Blagden is a Senior Lecturer in Forensic Psychology and Associate Head of the Sexual Offences Crime and Misconduct Research Unit at Nottingham Trent University (UK). He is a Chartered Psychologist and has worked and researched within the criminal justice system and HM Prison Service for many years.

Michelle Dwerryhouse is a PhD student at Nottingham Trent University, UK. She spent some time working in corporate business before completing her undergraduate degree in Psychology at the Open University in 2015. She then completed an MSc in Forensic Psychology and Mental Health at the University of Manchester in 2016. Michelle volunteered at Childline and Circles of Support and Accountability whilst studying, and worked with a prison mental health team during her MSc. She is currently working with the Safer Living Foundation to carry out a National Evaluation of Circles of Support and Accountability. Her research interests include offender rehabilitation and reintegration.

Kim Cox is a forensic psychologist in training. She did her undergraduate degree in Psychology with Neuroscience followed by a master's degree in Forensic Psychology. Kim has worked with Her Majesty's Prison and Probation Service (HMPPS) for over ten years and she specialises in the rehabilitation and risk assessment of people in prison for sexual offending.

Helen Elliott is a Lecturer in Counselling at Bishop Grosseteste University (UK). She has a background in forensic psychology with a focus on offender rehabilitation and therapeutic change and is a trainee integrative psychotherapist. Helen was also co-founder of the Safer Living Foundation—a charity set up to run rehabilitative initiatives.

Claire Good has spent the last 14 years working in the crime and community safety field, since gaining an MSc in Criminology. Most notably prior to her appointment as Young Persons Project Manager for the Safer Living Foundation she spent 8 years as a Manager within a Youth Offending Team with particular responsibility for work around victims, restorative justice, volunteers, referrals orders and prevention and early intervention.

Craig A. Harper is a Lecturer in Human Psychology at Nottingham Trent University (UK). His research interests lie in the psychological processes that underpin decision-making in relation to controversial social and political topics. Most of his research has been focused on how people form and express attitudes towards people with sexual convictions, with the aim being to promote progressive and evidence-based policies to prevent and reduce sexual victimisation. Away from forensically-based research, he is a member of the Heterodox Academy, which is an organisation seeking to promote viewpoint diversity and reduce political polarisation in higher education.

Dr Kerensa Hocken is a registered forensic psychologist at HMPPS Whatton (UK) and is an expert in the field of sexual offending. She has oversight for the assessment and treatment of people in prison for sexual offending in the Midlands region and is a co-founder, trustee and clinical lead for the Safer Living Foundation.

Rosie Kitson-Boyce has previously completed a BA in Criminology followed by an MSc in Psychology. Rosie has also worked as a psychology assistant in the prison service for 3 years where she facilitated on Sex offender treatment programmes. Following this Rosie completed an MSc in Forensic Psychology before starting a PhD at Nottingham Trent University. Rosie is currently completing her PhD, which is evaluating a prison-model of Circles of Support and Accountability. This research is part of the Sex Offences Crime and Misconduct Research Unit at the university. Rosie's research interests include, offender reintegration, rehabilitation and offenders with intellectual disabilities.

Rebecca Lievesley is a Lecturer in Forensic Psychology and member of the Sexual Offences, Crime and Misconduct Research Unit at NTU. She is also a co-founder and Trustee of the Safer Living Foundation.

Helen O'Connor is a trainee forensic psychologist who specialises in the field of sexual offending. She helped design and deliver the first group-based treatment programmes for deaf prisoners in HMPPS.

Dave Potter was born in England and has lived his whole life in the UK. He is a coordinator for the Safer living Foundations circles of support and accountability and has been working within the criminal justice system since 1989. He has extensive knowledge of sex offender treatment programmes and is especially interested in the rehabilitation back into the community of those convicted of sexual offences. He is committed to raising the profile of the work done by the SLF and he lives with his wife Susan, a teacher, and their 2 cats.

Carrie Webb is a qualified Probation Officer who worked in both community and custodial settings for a number of years prior to joining Circles South East in 2008 as the Circle Co-ordinator for Hampshire. Webb has been a Senior Co-ordinator since 2014 and has overall responsibility for the delivery of Circles across Hampshire, Surrey and Sussex. During the last four years she has overseen the design, implementation and delivery of the Adapted Circles pilot for individuals with learning disabilities and/or autism.

Chris Wilson is a qualified Social worker. He worked in Child Protection prior to his appointment as treatment manager at the Thames Valley Sex Offender Project. He was a member of the design team for the accredited Thames Valley Community Sex Offender Group-work Programme and in 2002 was appointed project manager for the Thames Valley Circles of Support and Accountability pilot project.

Belinda Winder is Head of the Sexual Crime, Misconduct and Research Unit at Nottingham Trent University (UK). She is a trustee, Vice Chair and co-founder of the Safer Living Foundation, a charity set up to prevent and reduce sexual offending.

List of Figures

Fig. 3.1	Recidivism rates taken from Wilson et al. (2007a, 2009)	46
Fig. 5.1	Representation of Maslow's hierarchy of needs	111
Fig. 8.1	Creative tools to help young people engage with a circle	183

List of Tables

Table 4.1 Core Member participant information 79
Table 4.2 Time point of data collection with Core Members 80
Table 4.3 Planned and actual number of prison CoSA sessions 80
Table 4.4 Themes from the interview data with corresponding data collection time points 81
Table 5.1 Dynamic risk domains 109

1

A History of the Development of Circles of Support and Accountability

Chris Wilson

The Historical Emergence and the International Spread of CoSA

In 2014, exactly twenty years after the first Circle of Support and Accountability (CoSA) had been established, over two hundred representatives from twenty-four countries gathered at the Cosmo Caixa in Barcelona, as the founding father of CoSA took to the stage to open the first international CoSA conference. In 1994, the Reverend Harry Nigh and a small number of volunteers from his congregation in the town of Hamilton (Ontario, Canada), offered support and protection to a lifelong recidivist child sex offender, known as Charlie Taylor. He told the conference of how this support was not without personal consequences, as public fear and panic, fuelled by a high-profile media campaign at Charlie's release from prison, led to threats of personal violence and damage to property. The courage and mediation shown by those volunteers, who became known as Charlie's Angels, created a better way of ensuring the

C. Wilson (✉)
Cardiff University, Cardiff, UK

H. Elliott et al. (eds.), *Sexual Crime and Circles of Support and Accountability*, Sexual Crime, https://doi.org/10.1007/978-3-319-74823-8_1

protection of children in a community that became Charlie Taylor's home until his death in 2011. The story of Charlie Taylor and the first CoSA is extensively documented (Wilson, Cortoni, & McWhinnie, 2009; Wilson, McWhinnie, & Wilson, 2008) and for many at that event in Barcelona, it was a story they knew well. Yet it remained a profoundly moving moment for all, to hear the story directly from the Reverend Nigh himself. He told of how Charlie had been institutionalised all his life, subjected to the care system as a child and then the prison system as an adult. A man with an intellectual disability who, prior to his CoSA was never able to sustain any prolonged period of release from prison before reoffending. The conference was also reminded of the courage needed when conviction requires action and that action is contrary not only to prevailing public opinion but the opinion of the statutory agencies charged with the risk management of individuals convicted of a sexual offence. He told how the CoSA had to navigate the complexities of a risk management model that at times would appear devoid of compassion and care. In an attempt to reduce Charlie's sense of isolation and loneliness, the CoSA volunteers had supported his acquisition of a cat, believing that caring for a living creature would give Charlie a focus and purpose, a sense of responsibility that would generally improve his well-being. The statutory agencies however could not see beyond Charlie's new pet as a means to entice children for the purpose of sexual offending, insinuating that the volunteers were being complicit in their support and advocacy of his ownership of a cat. What is significant and discussed later in this chapter, is that within a period of a decade the prevailing theoretical orthodoxy as how best to manage the risk of someone like Charlie had moved significantly from that of control, which focused upon criminogenic factors, to that which centred around personal agency and factors relating to the desistance of further reoffending. The story of Charlie's cat was certainly a timely reminder to the conference of the restorative nature of CoSA, and that common sense, humanity and care were the more likely ingredients that would help Charlie desist from further offending. This is a perspective now shared by many criminal justice professionals who have worked collaboratively with CoSA and is evidenced by Thomas when he states, "The CoSA model was considered a good model by all stakeholders and was seen as adding an extra dimension to the work that they themselves could do with sex offenders. However, CoSA also offered something different from the professional's contribution. There was broad agreement that the use of volunteers is good and volunteers were regarded positively by all respondents. Many of the stakeholders noted the levels of commitment displayed by the volunteers and the common-sense views which volunteers could bring to the role, which is unencumbered by professional training" (Thomas, Thompson, & Karstedt, 2014, p. 18).

Those persons fortunate enough to have been part of that first international conference held in Barcelona were able to celebrate a truly international movement with projects now established across Canada, Europe, the United States of America, Australia, New Zealand, South Africa, China and Japan, making CoSA one of the best known "restorative based reintegrative schemes for sex offenders" (McAlinden, 2007, p. 168).

Mennonite History Behind CoSA

Building upon a historic tradition by the Canadian Mennonites of facilitating restorative projects, including work specifically focused upon the use of community support in cases of sexual harm, CoSA became part of that tradition when a Mennonite Pastor, the Reverend Harry Nigh originally conceived of the concept. Its success led to the Mennonite Central Committee supporting the development of CoSA as a community reintegration project based upon restorative principles.

The Mennonite's historic tradition of such work within the criminal justice system was born in 1974 from a restorative experiment in Kitchener, Ontario, Canada, initially facilitated by Mark Yantzi, a probation officer from the Kitchener probation office. The experiment was essentially one of victim-offender mediation, whereby the victim was actively encouraged to be involved in decisions relating to reparation and restitution. Known as the Victim /Offender Reconciliation Project (VORP), it was immediately supported by both the local courts and the probation service. However, its development was greatly influenced by the thinking of the Norwegian criminologist Nils Christie (1977) and his assertion that the state had stolen people's conflict and was monopolising the criminal justice system. The importance of Christie's influence was the way in which the VORP attempted to de-professionalise the system by using community volunteers to undertake both the casework and facilitation of victim-offender mediation. It is at this point in the Mennonite tradition that the structural differences between the earlier Canadian and later British and European development of CoSA can be identified, in that, for the latter, the coordination of each CoSA, volunteer supervision and agency liaison remained with professionally qualified and paid staff.

By 1982, VORP began to develop and deliver additional victim services designed to support those who were victims of rape and incest. This work was again supported by Mennonite Central Committee and led to the creation of the Victim Services Programme which, over a number of years developed a raft of restorative and communitarian based services for those people whose lives had been blighted by sexual abuse, including direct work with individuals convicted of a sexual offence. These services included sexual offending treatment programmes, working with the partners of those individuals convicted of a sexual offence and the use of community volunteers to create networks of support for those individuals released from prison and returning to their families. The foundations therefore had been laid for the Mennonite Central Committee to give unequivocal support to the Reverend Harry Nigh and his congregation when, a decade later he and others like him would seek the Committee's support in the development of CoSA.

The timing of the first CoSA in Hamilton Ontario, coincided with a notable and significant change in public perceptions and hardening of attitudes towards those who committed sexual offences, particularly those who committed offences against children; the latter being regarded as the most loathsome group of all offenders. It was the recognition of such that led the Reverend Harry Nigh to conceive of the need for a community of care that would not only hold Charlie accountable, but also protect a community becoming increasingly fearful and intolerant of such offenders. Like Canada, the climate of public concern in the UK at the turn of the new millennium, created by a number of high profile cases of child abduction, sexual assault and murder had turned that concern into a tangible fear, resulting in numerous incidents of public disorder. CoSA, based as it was on restorative principles and community engagement spoke to the Quaker conscience who, in the United Kingdom took the Canadian experience direct to the British government, as a way of addressing the terror felt by someone who evokes such fear amongst a community to which they must return, and a way in which the community's fear could be addressed.

Development of CoSA in the UK

It was five years after the creation of Charlie's CoSA in Canada that the Quakers became aware of CoSA. Like Canada, Britain was experiencing a moral panic relating to child sexual abuse, fuelled by media campaigns such as the News of the Worlds 'Name and Shame'. For the Quakers, CoSA represented a peace project that had the ability to offer communities a restorative alternative to the fear generated by such campaigns. It was the Quakers that brought CoSA to the attention of the Home Office.

The Home Office had recently had to deal with the resettlement arrangements for Sydney Cooke and Robert Oliver, two notorious paedophiles who, with others had been involved in the sexual abuse of a young male, resulting in the victim's death. The continued media interest in Cooke and Oliver's release from prison combined with the subsequent public anger that they should not have been released at all, had made the Home Office all too aware of the increasing difficulty in safely managing the release and resettlement of high profile child sex offenders. This awareness resulted in the Home Office welcoming the chance to explore the feasibility of CoSA and, in June 2000, they invited key professionals to meet with colleagues from Canada. For the Home Office, the timing of this meeting was perfect; not only was it self-evident that CoSA would be wholly complementary in supporting the Home Office's newly instigated Multi Agency Public Protection Arrangements (MAPPA), a system in which those statutory agencies charged with the risk management of individuals convicted of a violent or sexual offence were required by law to meet on a regular basis, share information and formulate a risk management plan, but the philosophy and values of CoSA sat firmly within the government's Criminal Justice and Civil Renewal agendas that were central to the then, newly created National Offender Management Service known as NOMS (which, as of 2017, became Her Majesty's Prison and Probation Service or HMPPS).

All those involved in the meeting held at the Home Office in June 2000 were in agreement that the value of community involvement, as exampled through the work and evaluation (Wilson, Picheca, & Pinzo, 2005), of CoSA in Canada, was likely to be mutually beneficial to statutory agencies and staff alike in England. This was to be the starting point for the Home Office's funding of three separate pilot sites, two of which would be located geographically in Hampshire and the Thames Valley with the third pilot project to have a national remit, delivered by the Lucy Faithfull Foundation. The Foundation was a child protection charity who were running the only non-custodial residential sex offender treatment programme in the United Kingdom and whose residents would relocate anywhere in the country.

The ability of the Lucy Faithfull Foundation to respond to a request from any part of the country offered a different model of service delivery from the other two Home Office funded pilot projects. After a period of a decade, the Foundation had set up 36 CoSA which, given the logistical and geographical difficulties, was an outstanding achievement. However, the success and growth of CoSA nationally, required them to become geographically based. This they did, establishing a partnership with the West Midlands Probation area, close to their administrative headquarters in Alverchurch near Birmingham.

The Quaker's choice of geographical location for their pilot project, proved to be an astute strategy and played no small part in the project's success. There existed a history of restorative based practice amongst both police and probation in the Thames Valley with probation having developed one of three national accredited sex offender treatment programmes. The Thames Valley therefore appeared to be an area of fertile ground in which to grow a restorative based initiative such as CoSA.

The final government funded pilot project was Hampshire but by the end of the second year of government funding (2004), Hampshire was struggling. The Home Office impressed with Thames Valley, who during the same period of time had set up a total of 18 CoSA, asked Quakers to breathe new life into the Hampshire project and, within a year, a further six CoSA were operational.

During this same period, other CoSA projects, additional to those funded by the Home Office began to develop. In 2004, Greater Manchester's Community Chaplaincy received a small amount of Home Office funding following Hampshire CoSA being subsumed by Thames Valley. That same year the Prison Service secured European funding to deliver a project named, 'Innovation Means Prisons and Communities' (IMPACT). A project based at Young Offenders' Institution (YOI) Thorncross Warrington, focussed primarily on enhancing the employability of ex-offenders and using the CoSA model for those prisoners convicted of a sexual offence. IMPACT delivered a total of six successful CoSA in the Lancashire and Cheshire probation regions between 2004 and 2007 (Haslewood-Pocsik, Smith, & Spencer, 2008).

While in Northern Ireland, Robert Webb, a community worker inspired by the Canadian model, set up six CoSA between the years of 2003 and 2007. It should be remembered that the Good Friday Agreement had only been signed some five years previously and, both Webb and the volunteers he recruited demonstrated an enormous amount of courage engaging in such a project, set against a history of paramilitary activity and sectarian violence. In Scotland too, there existed a multi-agency development group. A feasibility study undertaken by Strathclyde University to test the viability of CoSA in Scotland (Armstrong, Chistyakova, Mackenzie, & Malloch, 2008), led to the Scottish government contributing to a pilot scheme in Fife (Armstrong & Wills, 2014). This eventually led to the roll out of CoSA across Scotland in the summer of 2014.

CoSA as a Restorative Model

Implicit in creating the context for the delivery of CoSA, the Quaker project set out to ensure practice was delivered within a sound theoretical framework. This framework needed to represent the understanding and values underpinning the CoSA model. The assertion that the model is a representation of community needs careful consideration. CoSA defines the notion of community in restorative terms as a collective of interconnected individuals who are all of equal importance. Implicit in that definition is the concept of mutual responsibility and the belief that people are accountable to one another. It is this accountability that characterises a community's interconnectedness and requires accountability to be "not just a passive responsibility but an active dynamic which sustains the welfare and happiness of others" (Hanvey, Philpot, & Wilson, 2011, p. 61). Such a perspective gives a deep resonance to the restorative principle that an injury to one is an injury to all. CoSA directly addresses this principle by facilitating the positive reintegration of the offender, known in CoSA as the Core Member back into the community, a perspective supported by Katherine Fox when she wrote, "Active civic engagement between offenders and citizens teaches community values explicitly via interactions designed to guide and support offenders as they transition (Bazemore & Stinchcomb, 2004). In addition, community values are transmitted implicitly by expressing the values of inclusion, citizenship, fundamental human rights, and forgiveness" (Fox, 2014, p. 5). When these values are applied to practice, there is a significant change in the way that justice is being delivered. This change is conceptualised by Kay Pranis (2007) as transformative, asserting that any values that support restorative practice have to be rooted in the two values of humanity and respect. Tim Newell (2007) applies Pranis' concept of transformation directly to the practice of CoSA. According to Newell, the success of CoSA as a truly restorative initiative can be measured by its compliance with the three principles:

> "The principle of repair—justice requires that we work to heal victims, offenders and communities that have been injured through crime (the work with offenders and helping them build their communities has been motivated by the need to avoid any further victims. Many of the volunteers who make up the COSAs are survivors of abuse). The principle of stakeholder participation—victims, offenders and communities should have the opportunity for active involvement in the justice process as fully as possible. The principle of transformation in community and government roles and relationships—This principle is well demonstrated in COSA's work where the community has taken much responsibility in exercising accountability and has been trusted by the agencies to work in this way". (Newell, 2007, p. 137)

Because there is no single agreed definition of Restorative Justice, it is best viewed as a patchwork of practice that articulates certain values (Ward, Fox, & Garber, 2014). These values then inform a process that facilitates all relevant stakeholders involved or affected by a crime, being able to express their feelings and needs in relation to any outcomes. The articulation of those values that support this need is what defines a practice as restorative. Pranis states that, "When people experience respect, equality and mutual care, they become more likely to drop defences or protections, which are often the source of destructive or non-cooperative behaviour. They become open to recognising common ground and acting in the common interest, a critical aspect of community" (Pranis, 2007, p. 68). It is the use of, and focus upon community rather than the process of individual victim offender conferencing or mediation that sets CoSA apart from other restorative practices and defines it as transformational. The paradox in relation to the transformational nature of CoSA is of course, its partnership and support of those very same agencies whose role restorative justice would seek to redefine. However, a number of commentators including Kathleen Daly (2003) have challenged the notion that restorative justice and retributive justice are incompatible and there is much evidence that the two do co-exist and are not mutually exclusive. This is particularly true for CoSA in that it shares the underlying restorative values of humanity and respect, is transformative in its active engagement of community and yet plays an important role, not only in relation to the application and delivery of rehabilitation but also in its support for the statutory sectors role in relation to the risk management of the Core Member, which clearly follows a retributive model of justice.

The Theoretical Framework

The theoretical framework (Saunders & Wilson, 2003) was based on three key principles. 'Support, Monitor and Maintain' and represented the adaptation of the Canadian model, into three distinct structures relating to the work undertaken by the statutory agencies. These three distinct principles also represent the three primary models of criminal justice, restorative, retributive and rehabilitative. 'Support' represents a restorative model, through inclusion, modelling and empathic concern. 'Monitor' represents a retributive model, highlighting MAPPA's need to maintain a risk averse stance and good systems of control, while CoSA offers MAPPA the ability to enhance public protection through the promotion of positive risk strategies that also have a rehabilitative measure for the Core Member. 'Maintain' represents a rehabilitative model, where CoSA works within a Risk, Needs and Responsivity framework, identifying criminogenic factors that can then be addressed through positive community reintegration using rehabilitative models such as the Good Lives Model (Ward & Stewart, 2003).

Each key principle contains a subset of principles relating to the desistance of sexual offending and enhancement of public protection. Accountability, through a relationship of support, lies at the heart of all healthy relationships and remains the central tenet of why CoSA are so effective. Acknowledging that high levels of emotional loneliness and isolation are two significant factors in recidivist behaviour, CoSA will seek to reduce these through the promotion of positive healthy relationships and do this by using the community in a transformational way. Perceptions of intimacy and deficits in attachments are addressed by the volunteers through appropriate modelling and are there to reinforce the moral norms of the community's own values.

By definition, the MAPPA process and subsequent actions tend to be reactive methods of control such as registration, sex offender prevention orders (SOPO) and community notification. CoSA afford this process the opportunity to facilitate a positive risk agenda whilst retaining the ability to gain intelligence without compromising the relationship between the offender and volunteers. Evidence accrued from practice highlights that Core Members continue to share problematic behaviours with their volunteers, knowing that any issue of risk will be communicated through the MAPPA process. The Core Member knowing this and still having a continued willingness to disclose information is evidence as to the viability of positive community involvement and as such, "monitoring becomes a constructive community based activity" (Carich, Wilson, Carich, & Calder, 2010, p. 203). Finally, the volunteers work to develop the Core Member's strategies to avoid reoffending previously identified through sex offender treatment. The purpose of CoSA, in its purest form, is to provide the Core Member with a support network so that the attempt to sustain a balanced, self-determined lifestyle becomes meaningful. It is in this way that the Core Member can acquire the mechanisms needed to achieve a positive life. The Core Member is only likely to accept the duality of support with accountability, if it is delivered within a context of humanity and care. This duality is evidenced when examining the Thames Valley's first CoSA, a referral that came directly from the Home Office.

The referral was a man named Peter, who had been assessed as high risk and predatory. He had a long history of sexually abusing children, including offences of child abduction and rape. He was to be released from prison having served a custodial sentence for the breach of a Sex Offender Prevention Order (SOPO) and had, at the bequest of the Home Office, agreed to be electronically tagged and reside in an Approved Probation Hostel. The Home Office, aware that they were providing funding for the newly established CoSA project, contacted the project manager and requested that CoSA be provided. Peter had never had any treatment, due to low intellectual functioning and remained in partial denial about much of his offending behaviour. His desire to desist from further offending appeared questionable and the risk that Peter posed was considered so serious that a previous psychologist's report had expressed the fear that future offending could lead to the death of a child. Despite reservations as to his suitability for CoSA, the decision was made that it was in everybody's interests that a CoSA be provided and Peter's profile seemed similar to that of Charlie, the recipient of Canada's first CoSA, which had proved successful some eight years previously. It was also reassuring that the British system, unlike Canada, was able to coordinate through MAPPA, a multi-agency post release plan on a person who was not subject to any statutory supervision.

Peter continued to be bound by the terms of his SOPO and was required to continue to fulfil the requirements of sex offender registration. The hostel in which Peter was accommodated, helped to develop a 'Through the Gate' model of CoSA practice, albeit from a probation hostel rather than a prison. This allowed Peter's CoSA volunteers to develop a relationship with him whilst he was still subject to the monitoring and support of a controlled environment. Such a model has since been developed within the prison system, both in the UK and Europe and facilitates a seamless transfer from incarceration into a community of care, which provides a function of intense support and monitoring. The support and help of both the hostel's management and staff was crucial in ensuring the early success of the CoSA's work with Peter.

Given the very high risk status of Peter, it was important that the volunteers in this CoSA were as diverse and robust as possible. The CoSA's work paid dividends in helping facilitate his access to part time employment, with later success in supporting his move from the probation hostel into sheltered accommodation.

Prior to the housing association agreeing to accommodate Peter, a risk management meeting was held and attended by managers from the association. Initially reluctant to agree to provide accommodation, the association's position changed after hearing about and meeting with representatives from Peter's CoSA. The warden of the accommodation, a survivor of sexual violence herself, was impressed and suggested that the association should accept Peter on a trial basis and that she too would undertake the CoSA training and become part of Peter's CoSA. The benefit of this arrangement was self-evident, with the warden not only being able to monitor the comings and goings from Peter's accommodation, but also offer support and communication through the CoSA network. The importance of this was demonstrated when Peter attempted to befriend a small group of school children, suggesting to them that they let him look after their youngest sibling.

By this time, the CoSA volunteers had worked with Peter for approximately eighteen months and over that period had observed positive changes in his self-esteem, confidence and personal hygiene. He had also begun to talk to the volunteers about his past offending and was acknowledging issues that he had previously denied. However, with the growth of Peter's confidence, came complacency and the volunteers began to detect renewed manipulation and deceptive behaviour replicating issues evident in his previous offending. The discovery by the CoSA volunteers of Peter's attempts to groom a group of children precipitated an immediate recall, again on a voluntary basis, back to the Probation hostel for both his own and the public's protection. The children were interviewed by the Police and while no report of a sexual assault was made, Peter was arrested and bailed to reside at the hostel. The Crown Prosecution Service decided that it would not pursue a charge of grooming but he was charged once for breach of his SOPO. Upon sentencing, the Court concluded that the CoSA had prevented a serious further offence taking place and sentenced Peter to a three year Community Sentence order with a condition of residence back at the Probation hostel, allowing the work of the CoSA to continue.

This particular case serves as an example of how, even with the most difficult of people, the restorative concept of transformation can be successfully applied. Peter remained part of CoSA for a further eight years during which time, he was never convicted of a further sexual offence. However, his repeated breach of the SOPO demonstrated the continuous tension between the rights of the individual and the need for good public protection, which have to be managed by both the statutory agencies and CoSA volunteers alike. However, the ability of the CoSA volunteers to address Peter's criminogenic factors not only shows the restorative transformational element of CoSA but also its ability to positively implement strength based rehabilitative theory into practice.

CoSA as a Rehabilitative Model

It could be argued that it was the application of the rehabilitation model to the development of CoSA in the United Kingdom that set it apart from the Canadian model. The initial criteria for Core Member referral implemented by the Thames Valley CoSA pilot project was based upon the Core Member being subject to the MAPPA and having completed the accredited Thames Valley Sex Offender Treatment Programme, a programme based upon the Risk Needs Responsivity (RNR) model (Andrews & Bonta, 1998). Although evidenced based, the model continues to support the prevailing orthodoxy of control. The primary criticism of this model in relation to reducing recidivism is that it neglects both personal agency and identity relating to any process of change and its focus upon criminogenic factors fails to recognise the relevance of the therapeutic alliance, a key factor in the change process (Mann & Shingler, 2006). It also ignores the importance of the offender's environment and social context, which often contribute to dynamic risk (Ward & Maruna, 2007).

This is where CoSA proved to be so successful in that it functioned within the Core Member's environment and was relational, thereby facilitating a therapeutic alliance. CoSA's rehabilitative nature was further enhanced through its practice of the Core Member sharing with their volunteers the work completed in treatment and the content of their relapse prevention plan based upon the Good Lives Model (Ward & Stewart, 2003). This facilitated the volunteers performing the dual role of supporting the implementation of the relapse prevention plan, while also being aware of the Core Member's criminogenic factors, high risk situations, triggers and coping strategies. In this way, the volunteers were also able to hold the Core Member accountable. However, a study commissioned by Circles UK in 2014 and undertaken by Leeds University, identified what appeared to be confusion amongst CoSA volunteers regarding their interpretation and meaning related to the role of holding the Core Member accountable. The identification of what the report referred to as "a lack of a defined and collective understanding of this central concept" (Thomas, Thompson, & Karstedt, 2014, p. 17) was important and had significant implications for national volunteer policies and training. Despite the deficit of a shared understanding, the report was able to identify that the volunteers were holding Core Members to account as well as successfully effecting some changes in their behaviour. It is of interest that the study highlighted that while the volunteers were clear regarding the role of support, the meaning of accountability was more ambiguous. Whether this finding was a result of the development of the British CoSA model trying to combine two separate justice models, restorative and rehabilitative, remains a matter of conjecture. It does however highlight the tension that exists between the two concepts of support and accountability. Despite this tension, CoSA does appear to be able to bridge the divide between its restorative, transformational nature and the rehabilitative role it was designed to deliver. It has achieved this due to the shared values and similar theoretical underpinnings of both the rehabilitative and restorative theories. "Rehabilitation theory is essentially a hybrid theory comprised of values, principles, etiological assumptions and practice guidelines. In effect, it contains elements of normative, etiological and practice/treatment theories within it while being broader than just the sum of its parts" (Ward & Maruna, 2007, p. 33).

The late 1990s had seen a significant development in rehabilitative theory influencing models of practice and academics and practitioners alike had begun to ask the question, not 'What Works?' but 'What helps?' Reframing the question in this way was to "shift the focus away from criminogenic need and other deficits and instead ask what the individual can contribute to his or her family, community and society" (Ward & Maruna, 2007, p. 23). This shift in perspective was known as the strength based approach and required those working with offenders to distinguish that which is "desistance-focused from that which is offending related" (McNeil, 2006, p. 46). Although it had always been the aim of rehabilitative intervention to prevent reoffending, previous theories and practice as typified by the RNR model reinforced the negative, by targeting the individual's deficits and managing them as a set of risk factors. In contrast to this, a desistance-focused strength based approach works towards that which is positive, increasing the individual's investment in social capital and therefore achieving a successful reintegration into the wider community. During the development of the Government funded CoSA pilot projects, the Good Lives Model, a strength based theory, had been introduced into Sex Offender Treatment Programmes and was being delivered in both prisons and the community. Good Lives is a psychological model that is desistance-focused and is based upon two fundamental aims. First, it identifies and promotes those basic needs that all of us require to have a satisfying and fulfilling life, these basic needs are referred to as 'human goods' and second, it aims to provide those offenders with the skills needed to achieve the acquisition of those 'human goods'. The reality is that the concept and theory of the model delivered in a treatment group remains just that, conceptual and theoretical. What treatment facilitators, probation staff and MAPPA managers all recognised was that CoSA's delivery could embody the model, making it dynamic. It facilitated the Core Member's ability to practice the skills needed within the community and to successfully achieve those goals previously identified during treatment. The model gives resonance to four prerequisites identified by Braithwaite (1989) for successful reintegration. Condemnation of the crime rather than of the offender, a prerequisite that is essential for CoSA volunteers to follow and a principle that is the essence of the Good Lives Model, "offenders are essentially human beings with similar needs and aspirations to non-offending members of the community" (Ward & Stewart, 2003, p. 43). Secondly, the need to maintain a relationship of respect between the Core Member and the volunteers. Thirdly, the work of CoSA is undertaken within a context of approval and acceptance, overtly demonstrated through the support of the volunteers and the professional 'Outer Circle' and finally, reintegration is marked with ceremonies of forgiveness and acceptance, which McAlinden described the CoSA as achieving. "The net result is the sex offender receives sympathy and help in reintegration and not just hostility, from at least some members of the community" (McAlinden, 2007, p. 173)

Ministerial Support for CoSA

The response to CoSA from the professional agencies, combined with its success in recruiting and sustaining an ever-growing volunteer base, facilitated a growing confidence from the government, that led to the funding of three pilot sites. They could now begin to evidence the benefits of CoSA upon the risk management of sex offenders being released into the community. This confidence was demonstrated when Jane Griffiths, MP for Reading East, secured a short House of Commons debate focussed on the work of CoSA. Paul Goggins, a minister of state based at the Home Office, who had previously given a keynote address at the first national CoSA conference held at Friends House in London on the 7 July 2004, affirmed the government's commitment to CoSA and later the same day spoke on the subject in parliament. He confirmed that the Home Office were already providing £173,000 to fund CoSA pilots with almost half of that money going to the Thames Valley CoSA project. Although an evaluation was awaited he was able to report that:

> "I am pleased with the initial feedback that I have received from the earliest circles, which includes a range of evidence on such matters as offenders being supported in a way that enables them to live more independently, by getting a job, for example, or moving to their own accommodation, thereby helping them to overcome personal crises that are, perhaps, inevitable after a long period in prison". (Hansard HC Debates, 7 July 2004)

Circles UK

It was the beginning of the new millennium when the British government invested in CoSA and they did so in the context of what appeared to be a moral panic related to child sex offenders. Once established and operating, the interest was immediate, with CoSA being a consistent and high-profile topic at all MAPPA Conferences the length and breadth of the country. This interest, combined with the encouraging early results from the Canadian evaluations, led to the development of a number of other CoSA projects across England and Wales. The intervening years between Paul Goggins' speech in Parliament in 2004 and the advent of Circles UK in 2008 saw the development of a further six projects across both England and Wales. These new projects did not have the luxury of direct government funding and were looking to their local police and probation areas for support both operationally and financially. This income was successfully supplemented by various philanthropic trusts, who were inspired by the concept of CoSA and its successful implementation.

However, the speed of these developments gave rise to concern and an assurance was needed by the British government that the new projects would operate within the parameters of best practice as developed by the pilot sites. Therefore, in 2005, the Home Office commissioned the Quakers to engage in a process of consultation as how best to achieve a consistent quality of practice. In 2007, with government funding from the then newly formed Ministry of Justice, a new independent charitable organisation was launched known as Circles UK.

This new charity was to be an 'umbrella' organisation that would operate a system of membership for all projects delivering CoSA. Its remit was to focus upon six key objectives (2008):

- *Development*, to develop the delivery of CoSA across England and Wales. It achieves this by supporting the coordination of information, advice and training to all its member projects;
- *Quality*, to ensure that there is a quality and consistency of practice in all work undertaken within a CoSA. This is achieved by providing a set

of standards relating to the training of both volunteers and CoSA coordinators and then developing and implementing a system of assessment against which the standards could be measured;
- *Evaluation and research*, Circles UK takes the lead with regard to national evaluation and research ensuring the facilitation of national forums that helps promote learning specifically related to CoSA practice;
- *Media*, Circles UK coordinates all media relations and act as a conduit to provide the media with accurate information about CoSA. This is done in conjunction with the promotion of public awareness and education;
- *Influence and promotion*, to influence the development of CoSA and maintain their profile with strategic partners (Police and Probation) at both a regional and national level;
- *Sustainability*, to ensure the sustainability of local CoSA projects and to support their expansion into mainstream activity by adopting a coordinated and high level approach to funding negotiations.

Various agencies, organisations and community groups across the country were now able to seek support from Circles UK in helping them establish the infrastructure for locally based CoSA projects. Although the Quakers had now relinquished direct involvement with CoSA, launching their original pilot project in the Thames Valley as an independent charity, known now as Circles South East, local Quaker groups felt an implicit sense of ownership and continued at local level to support CoSA through numerous practical ways. In 2007, Carlisle Quaker Meeting, through a bequest, established a CoSA project in Cumbria, while Quakers in Norwich sought to establish a project across the East of England.

Lynn Saunders, Governor of HMP Whatton also approached Circles UK requesting support and guidance as to the possibility to develop an adapted 'Through the Gate' model of CoSA, in which the volunteers would establish a relationship with the Core Member/prisoner prior to release. This was achieved through the creation of a charity known as the Safer Living Foundation and was unique in that integral to their model was a partnership with Nottingham Trent University. This type of partnership was to be the model that would be adopted for the further implementation of CoSA projects across Europe, funded by the European Commission.

By the end of 2010, Circles UK had produced a Code of Practice, against which all projects could ensure a sustainable and solid practice base and a process of membership, renewal and audit was developed to be measured against the code of practice criteria. Through its federation, the organisation supports, to date, 16 individual member projects spread across England and Wales, all of which are supported by their local police and probation area. Funding and media protocols were written in an attempt to ensure that no two projects are chasing the same pot of money and that there is a coordinated and structured response to all media enquiries. Circles UK has engaged in the commissioning and development of risk assessment tools and research programmes, as well as organising national coordinator training events and a number of annual conferences.

There are however two specific achievements that Circles UK can rightly be proud of. The first is its achievement in securing two and a quarter million pounds of funding from the National Lottery to develop CoSA in those areas of the UK currently without. The rationale for this was to ensure national coverage ready for possible commissioning by the National Probation Service. The other formidable achievement was the organisations role in the design, development and proliferation of CoSA across Europe, funded by the European Commission.

European CoSA

Nowhere has the growth of CoSA been more successful, specifically in terms of its coordination, implementation and sustained integration, than across the various European countries and jurisdictions.

The success and growth of CoSA in the UK and its relevance specifically to MAPPA, led to the Confederation of European Probation (CEP) actively promoting the concept through a conference it held in Glasgow 2008. It was this CEP conference that led to the first European Commission funded CoSA project 'Together in Safety', a consortium of partner agencies that included Circles UK, the Dutch and Belgium Probation Service, all supported by Avans University in Holland. This project not only successfully established CoSA in Holland and Belgium but also produced a manual for contextual consideration when implementing CoSA in other European jurisdictions. The European commission, impressed with the projects' outcomes, invited a further application to establish a second European Project that would roll out CoSA across a further six European countries.

This specific European Project known as Circles 4EU had three aims, firstly, to unify CoSA and to develop the European CoSA network for the purposes of training, guidance and support for all new European services, defining and setting the CoSA principles and values. Secondly, to ensure research which will oversee the objective of supporting and evaluating all identified work-streams, expanding the knowledge base to ensure maximum effectiveness and impact of CoSA across a wide set of national and geographical locations. And thirdly, supporting the establishment of the three new CoSA services in Catalonia, Latvia and Bulgaria, with a further three countries (France, Hungary and the Republic of Ireland), developing the infrastructure to implement in the future. The Republic of Ireland were able to successfully secure funding from the Probation Service that allowed them to achieve both the development of project infrastructure and operational viability. The Circles 4EU project culminated in November 2014 with an international conference hosted by the Catalonian Justice Department in Barcelona.

Conclusion

CoSA has become a truly international movement. It inspires policy makers, practitioners and members of the public alike, who recognise that inclusive and supportive engagement with persons known to have committed a sexual offence, will ultimately reduce further sexual offending (Bates, Williams, Wilson, & Wilson, 2013). CoSA's ability to support an individual in their desire to achieve an offence free future, does so within a humane and constructive environment. The adaptation of the original Canadian model into a British context facilitated CoSA's integration into the MAPPA and risk management process. This integration was only possible because, as a model, CoSA are able to integrate both restorative and rehabilitative theory. Despite a period of austerity due to a global economic downturn, the Canadian government have provided the Mennonite Central Committee with substantial funding for CoSA, 7.5 million dollars, from September 2009 to 2014 and then a further 7.48 million dollars in May 2017 (https://www.thestar.com/news/canada/2017/05/07/ottawa-gives-748m-for-sex-offender-reintegration-program.html). Over the past 10 years, the British government has part funded Circles UK and CoSA projects are now established across Europe, the United States of America, Australia and New Zealand.

The international growth of CoSA has created the opportunity for global collaboration in both practice and research. Collaboration will achieve a collective understanding of what needs to be in place to meet the justice needs of victims, offenders and their communities, giving substance to the original CoSA mantra of 'No More Victims'.

References

Andrews, D. A., & Bonta, J. (1998). *The psychology of criminal conduct.* Cincinnati, OH: Anderson.

Armstrong, S., Chistyakova, Y., Mackenzie, S., & Malloch, M. (2008). *Circles of support and accountability: Consideration of the feasibility of pilots in Scotland.* Report No. 1/2008, The Scottish Centre for Crime and Justice Research, Glasgow.

Armstrong, S., & Wills, D. (2014). Circles of support and accountability (COSA) in Scotland: Practice, progress and questions. *Scottish Journal of Criminal Justice Studies, 20*, 2–13.

Bates, A., Williams, D., Wilson, C., & Wilson, R. (2013). Circles South East: The first 10 years 2002–2012. *International Journal of Offender Therapy and Comparative Criminology, 58*, 861–885.

Bazemore, G., & Stinchcomb, J. (2004). A civic engagement model of re-entry: Involving community through service and restoration. *Federal Probation, 68*, 1–14.

Braithwaite, J. (1989). *Crime, shame and reintegration.* Cambridge University Press.

Carich, M., Wilson, C., Carich, P., & Calder, M. (2010). Contemporary sex offender treatment: Incorporating circles of support and the good lives model. In J. Brayford, F. Cowe, & J. Deering (Eds.), *What else works? Creative work with offenders* (pp. 188–210). Cullompton: Willan Publishing.

Christie, N. (1977, January). Conflicts as property. *The British Journal of Criminology, 17*, 1–5.

Circles UK. (2008). Code of Practice Version 1 (available from Circles UK Abbey House Reading RG1 3BE).

Daly, K. (2003). Restorative justice: The real story. In G. Johnstone (Ed.), *A restorative justice reader. Texts, sources, context* (p. 363). Willan Publishing.

Fox, K. J. (2014). Behavior theorizing community integration as desistance-promotion. *Criminal Justice and Behavior*. Published online 25 September 2014. https://doi.org/10.1177/0093854814550028. The online version of this article can be found at: http://cjb.sagepub.com/content/early/2014/09/25/0093854814550028

Hansard HC Debates. (7 July 2004). vol. 423 cc296305WH.

Hanvey, S., Philpot, T., & Wilson, C. (2011). *A community based approach to the reduction of sexual reoffending circles of support and accountability*. London: Jessica Kingsley Publishers.

Haslewood-Pocsik, I., Smith, E., & Spencer, J. (2008, January). *IMPACT circles: Balancing risk management with support: A study of an innovative approach in working with sex offenders*. Final report. University of Manchester, Manchester.

Mann, R., & Shingler, J. (2006). Collaboration in clinical work with sex offenders: Treatment and risk assessment. In W. L. Marshall, Y. E. Fernandez, L. E. Marshall, & G. A. Serran (Eds.), *Sexual offender treatment: Controversial issues*. Chichester: John Wiley.

McAlinden. (2007). *The shaming of individual convicted of a sexual offences risk, retribution and reintegration*. Hart Publishing.

McNeill, F. (2006). A desistance paradigm for offender management. *Criminology and Criminal Justice, 6*, 39–62.

Newell, T. (2007). *Forgiving justice: A Quaker vision for criminal justice Swarthmore Lecture 2000*. London: Quaker Books.

Pranis, K. (2007). Restorative values. In G. Johnstone & D. Van Ness (Eds.), *Handbook of restorative justice* (p. 68). Willan Publishing.

Saunders, R., & Wilson, C. (2003, July). Circles of support and accountability in the Thames Valley: Questions and answers. *NOTA News 45*.

Thomas, T., Thompson, D., & Karstedt, S. (2014). *Assessing the impact of circles of support and accountability on the reintegration of adults convicted of sexual offences in the community*. Final report. Centre for Criminal Justice Studies, School of Law, University of Leeds.

Ward, T., Fox, K. J., & Garber, M. (2014). Restorative justice, offender rehabilitation and desistance. *Restorative Justice, 2*(1), 24–42.
Ward, T., & Maruna, S. (2007). *Rehabilitation.* Oxon: Routledge.
Ward, T., & Stewart, C. (2003). Criminogenic needs and human needs: A theoretical model. *Psychology, Crime and Law, 9*, 125–143.
Wilson, R. J., Cortoni, F., & McWhinnie, A. W. (2009). Circles of support & accountability: A Canadian national replication of outcome findings. *Sexual Abuse: A Journal of Research and Treatment, 21*, 412–430.
Wilson, R. J., McWhinnie, A., & Wilson, C. (2008). Circles of support and accountability: An international partnership in reducing individual convicted of a sexual offence recidivism. *Prison Service Journal, 178*, 26–36.
Wilson, R. J., Picheca, J. E., & Pinzo, M. (2005). *Circles of support and accountability: An evaluation of the pilot project in South Central Ontario.* Research Report R. 168. Ottawa, ON: Correctional Service of Canada.

2

Circles of Support and Accountability, Assisted Desistance and Community Transition

Nicholas Blagden, Helen Elliott, and Rebecca Lievesley

Introduction

In the previous chapter, Chris Wilson outlined the historical and theoretical foundations of Circles of Support and Accountability (CoSA) and explicated the CoSA model. This chapter builds on the previous chapter and examines where CoSA fits within the desistance literature. Recent empirical research concerned with offender rehabilitation and reintegration has focused on what promotes desistance from crime. A central aspect of the desistance process is the transformation and changes in the narrative identity of crime desisters (Maruna, 2001). Desistance researchers argue that successful desistance hinges on internal promoters (such as narrative identity shift) and external promoters (such as employment and marriage). Furthermore, there has been a move within the literature to consider not just the risk and criminogenic needs of those who have com-

---

N. Blagden (✉) • R. Lievesley
Nottingham Trent University, Nottingham, UK

H. Elliott
Bishop Grosseteste University, Lincoln, UK

H. Elliott et al. (eds.), *Sexual Crime and Circles of Support and Accountability*, Sexual Crime, https://doi.org/10.1007/978-3-319-74823-8_2

mited sexual crime, but also to understand the process of desistance and the need for individuals to address protective factors, for example, positive self-identity (de Vries Robbé, Mann, Maruna, & Thornton, 2015). However, an under researched aspect of the desistance process is the role of community members in integrating released offenders back into the community (Fox, 2015). The aim of this chapter is to consider where COSA may fit in terms of the wider desistance literature and recent models of desistance.

CoSA are an intervention used with medium to very high risk individuals who have been convicted of a sexual offence. The aim is to support and enable their reintegration back into society, whilst still holding them accountable for their behaviour (Cesaroni, 2001) (see Chap. 1 for more detail). A Circle consists of three to six members of the local community who volunteer to meet weekly with the Core Member (the individual who has committed a sexual offence). Supervised by a project coordinator, a Circle aims to establish a pro-social network around the individual, providing practical and emotional support. There are several significant dimensions to community-based integration programmes like CoSA. First, the model illustrates the power of positive labelling in moving an offender from a state of temporal desistance to a more enduring identity (Fox, 2015). Indeed, there are inherent benefits from moving individuals away from the 'sex offender' label, as this can impair positive self-identity (see e.g. Blagden, Winder, & Hames, 2014; Maruna, 2001). Developing a sense of belonging and constructing desirable identities is important for the self-change process and ultimately for tertiary desistance (Farmer, Maruna, & McAlinden, 2016; McNeill, 2014). "As such, community integration can be seen as a precursor to successful desistance, rather than an outcome of desistance" (Fox, 2015, p. 91).

Desistance and CoSA

The concept of narrative identity is important for the rehabilitation and crime desistance of those convicted of sexual offences, as those lacking a coherent narrative identity are often thought more likely to continue to offend (Ward & Marshall, 2007). In the desistance literature, identity change/transformation has been linked to 'redemptive' episodes whereby the negative past self is reconstrued as positive because it has led to the transformation of that person; the past self is construed as qualitatively different from the changed self (McAdams, 2006b). Consequently, shifts in personal identity have been argued as important for desistance (Göbbels, Ward, & Willis, 2012). Such redemptive narratives can restore moral agency, in turn empowering the narrators to imagine and pursue generative futures. They allow for 'real selves' to be emphasised and for negative past incidents to be reconstrued as life experiences that made them stronger, wiser, better prepared for the future and wanting to give something back (Stone, 2015). Stone (2015) argues for the importance of identity-repairing narratives in the desistance process and the how the internalisation of oppressive master narratives may restrict opportunities for desistance. Thus, allowing offenders to enact/portray *good* selves can lead to *living* those roles as people tend to act in line with the stories they present about themselves (Blagden et al., 2014; Friestad, 2012; McAdams, 2006a).

This chapter will now turn to how CoSA fits within established models of desistance and how it may facilitate/assist with desistance. Given that desistance rests upon an interplay between structure and agency, the chapter will focus on CoSA's potential contribution to meaningful narrative and psychological change, the process of CoSA, that is the contribution of the relational dynamics to the desistance process, and how it reintegrates individuals with convictions for sexual offences back into the community.

CoSA, Narratives of Change and Identity Change

Göbbels et al. (2012) have emphasised the importance of positive practical identities in the desistance process and the importance of 'turning points' or constructive outlets which provide opportunities for the momentum of change in which the self is construed in a positive light. It may be that CoSA provide such possibilities and have the potential to assist with positive identity change as individuals transition from prison to the community. Indeed, research by Kitson-Boyce, Blagden, Winder, and Dillon (2016) highlights how prison CoSA can further bolster the traditional CoSA model by preparing individuals for release and bolstering their identity pre-release. LeBel, Burnett, Maruna, and Bushway (2008) found that self-identification and positive self-image were significant predictors of post-prison outcomes. In contrast, feelings of stigmatisation predicted reoffending (Chiricos, Barrick, & Bales, 2007).

Göbbels et al. (2012) formulated the Integrated Theory of Desistance from Sexual Offending (ITDSO). This is a four-stage theory describing the processes by which individuals with sexual crime convictions transition from incarceration to living a crime-free life. Phase one is labelled 'decisive momentum' and refers to the stage at which a former sexual offender makes a conscious decision that their offending behaviour is problematic and needs to stop. This occurs through processes of self-realisation, or as a result of some external catalyst (e.g. a new relationship, or changes in life circumstances). In phase two ('rehabilitation'), formal sexual offender rehabilitation procedures (e.g., prison-based Sex Offender Treatment Programmes) are introduced to focus on the successful "reconstruction of the self" (Göbbels et al., 2012, p. 457). The aim at this point of the desistance process is to provide support to those who want to change their sexual offending behaviour by helping them to develop the skills needed to do so through positive identity restructuring. It can be noted that CoSA fits well within this stage, as the relationships with volunteers not only provide support, but also nurture pro-social narratives. As Fox (2015) found, volunteers within CoSA encourage Core Members to reconstruct and maintain a more positive sense of self though the inclusive nature of the initiative. Phase three ('re-entry') highlights the importance of an external rehabilitation-reinforcing environment, within which people with convictions for sexual offences can begin to rebuild and maintain their new identities as non-offenders. The emphasis here is on maintaining the commitment to change, which requires the construction of a new, positive, non-offender identity achieved in the previous phase (Göbbels et al., 2012). CoSA volunteers have the opportunity to assist in this process by providing ongoing empathic support and encouragement to the Core Member, something Göbbels et al. (2012)

suggested can be achieved through mentoring. This is not always easy in a society where those who commit sexual crime are deemed as the worst of the worst (see Chap. 6 for a focus on attitudes towards sexual offenders). However, by the volunteers not only offering their own support, but encouraging Core Members to socialise outside of the Circle, this can reinforce and strengthen their new identity as a non-offender (Elliott & Zajac, 2015). Höing, Bogaerts, and Vogelvang (2013) found that the positive relationships and engagement in prosocial activities led to an increased motivation to build on this in their own social world. One Core Member in the study reported that he had shown more interest in others and that "expressing interest in others has proven to be a positive experience in the Circle" (p. 284). This finding is also supported within the findings of Kitson-Boyce where a Core Member described becoming less isolated and integrating more into society after experiencing the support within his CoSA. More on this can be read in Chap. 4 of this book. Finally, in phase four ('normalcy'), these individuals fully adopt this new identity, and view themselves as non-offenders. Stages 3 and 4 of the model focus more on the conditions necessary for successful identity change, that is social context and social relationships. This fourth phase would see the ending of CoSA for the Core Member, where meetings are reduced and eventually cease, as support from the volunteers is required less and less due to the adoption and integration of their new identity.

Göbbels et al. (2012) identified the importance of a rehabilitation-reinforcing social environment, such as the maintenance of positive social relationships and a strong non-offender identity. However, they also point out the difficulties associated with achieving these social conditions with a history of sexual offending, through the processes of stigmatization, labelling, and strict probation restrictions (Levenson & Cotter, 2005). Indeed, punitive social attitudes towards individuals with sexual crime convictions can interfere with the desistance process. There are paradoxical findings when examining community attitudes towards individuals with sexual crime convictions. For example, it has been found that 95% of people agreed that persons convicted of sex crime should receive therapy (Brown, 1999) and that 39–49% agreed that 'Society has an obligation to assist sex offenders released into the community to live better lives' (McAlinden, 2007). However, there are pervasive beliefs about the irredeemability of individuals with sexual crime convictions. For example, 23% of the public agreed that 'Most people who commit sexual offences against *adults* can go on to live law abiding lives', while 16% agreed that 'Most people who commit sexual offences against *children* can go on to live law abiding lives' (McAlinden, 2007). Moreover, 64% would oppose the locating of a treatment centre in their neighbourhood (Brown, 1999). Attitudes towards individuals with sexual crime convictions are important for the rehabilitative process (see Chap. 6 which explores this and media representation in more detail). Indeed, attitudes towards individuals with sexual crime convictions are important for the rehabilitative process and have been found to predict whether staff who work with such individuals have positive or punitive views towards their rehabilitation (Craig, 2005; Kjelsberg & Loos, 2008) and are associated with beliefs that offenders can change (Blagden et al., 2014). Importantly, attitudes towards individuals with sexual crime convictions have been linked to therapeutic effectiveness and therapeutic alliance.

Relational and Reciprocal Aspects of CoSA

Since desistance is about, in part, discovering agency, interventions need to encourage and respect self-determination; this means working with offenders, "not on them" (McCulloch, 2005). The importance of individuals convicted of crimes 'owning' their own rehabilitation, being invested in it or having a stake in it should not be underestimated. This has led some to argue that there is a need for offenders *to do* desistance and not just *talk* desistance (Blagden & Perrin, 2016). Given the emphasis that CoSA places on community integration, the relational exchanges between Core Members and volunteers and the dual process of emotional/pastoral support and accountability give rise to the conditions that allow for Core Members to 'own' or have a stake in their own rehabilitation. The relational aspects of CoSA have been found to assist with desistance-based narratives (see e.g. Fox, 2015) and could contribute to self-determination and 'active citizenship' (Perrin & Blagden, 2014). As previously highlighted, belonging to a group and encountering meaningful social relationships are crucial in the desistance process—it is rarely a solitary pursuit. Weaver and McNeill (2015) reported that the social relations that were most influential in supporting desistance were those characterised by a sense of belonging and solidarity. Desistance from crime, it appears, is much easier for those who are able to embed themselves within social networks, which support their new pro-social identities (Paternoster & Bushway, 2009). This links to a fundamental aspect of CoSA and points to the importance of the relational dynamics within Circles.

In an attempt to provide a theoretical underpinning to CoSA, Höing et al. (2013) interviewed Core Members and found that CoSA volunteers are able to provide exactly that which Weaver and McNeill described. Core Members felt a sense of togetherness, and it being about "all of us" (p. 278), rather than just focusing on the Core Member. Inclusion was identified as one of the essential functions of a successful CoSA in this study. As well as the more obvious inclusive functions of a Circle, such as the regular meetings and discussions about the Core Member's issues, some of the most meaningful elements of a Circle for the Core Member were the more generic discussions about both the volunteers' and Core Members' interests. In particular, the sharing of personal information from volunteers contributed to a greater "sense of belonging" and being part of a community once again (p. 283). This fits with the findings of Weaver and McNeill (2015), who demonstrated that the social relations most influential in supporting desistance are those categorised by a sense of 'we-ness', which in turn shapes a sense of belonging and reinforces the new pro-social identity.

There is a growing evidence base that relationships in correctional settings and supportive rehabilitative settings assist with the desistance process. So much so that the relationship between service user and practitioner has been reinstated as a core condition for changing both the social circumstances and behaviour associated with recidivism by policy-makers (Burnett & McNeill, 2005). This is in light of research demonstrating the impact that staff attitudes have on the success of rehabilitative interventions (Craig, 2005). The importance of the therapeutic relationship/working alliance however is not a new one, and has long been recognised as one of the most (if not the most) important factors influencing therapeutic change (Rogers, 1951; Horvath & Greenberg, 1989; Horvath

& Luborsky, 1993). Recent research demonstrates that the relational dynamics of staff-prisoner interactions is an important aspect in individuals' rehabilitation (Blagden & Perrin, 2016; Blagden, Perrin, Smith, Gleeson, & Gillies, 2017; Perrin & Blagden, 2014). Participants spoke of reciprocal relationships with both staff and fellow prisoners that were based on respect, mutual helping, and learning. These relational interactions appeared to represent a testing ground for relationship building post-prison. Indeed, establishing social relationships is vital in terms of triggering, enabling, and sustaining change (Weaver, 2015). One of the aims of CoSA is to foster companionship and trust between the Core Member and volunteers, something which is thought to be essential to successful reintegration (Youssef, Casey, & Birgden, 2017). The most effective reintegration is thought to be possible in communities where significant interpersonal relationships are many (Braithwaite, 1989).

Furthermore, Vaughan (2007) has argued that change narratives require continuous validation. Indeed, validation that change is recognised is important to the desistance process and that this change is not only recognised but reflected back to them. There is a body of research that highlights the importance of pygmalion effects (high expectation produces higher outcome) and interpersonal expectancy effects on prisoner outcomes (Maruna, 2004).

Maruna, LeBel, Naples, and Mitchell (2009) have argued that self-change occurs not only through self-appraisals and attributions but also from the reactions and reflected appraisals of others. In Tate, Blagden, and Mann (in press) the reciprocal nature of interactions within the prison constituted a source of validation for the prisoner participants. This again points to the relational properties in the 'self-change' process (Mead, Hilton, & Curtis, 2001). This validation process through reciprocal relationships is also something that is particularly important for individuals with sexual crime convictions who experience high levels of shame and stigma (Blagden, Winder, Thorne, & Gregson, 2011).

Sexual crime is often deemed the worst of the worst, and communities as a whole tend to view those who commit these crimes with hatred and fear (Petrunik, 2003). This can lead to stigmatisation and shaming of this group of individuals, something which increases the risk of an individual reoffending (Braithwaite, 1989). Braithwaite's (1989) theory of reintegrative shaming however, distinguishes between negative shaming (disintegrative) and good shaming (reintegrative). He explained how actively shaming the behaviour rather than the individual, coupled with forgiveness, acceptance and respect can help prevent sexual crime from occurring. Conversely, disintegrative shaming only serves to stigmatise and isolate, factors that increase the likelihood of reoffending. Thus, if the reactions and reflected appraisals of others are negative, self-change may be impaired or hindered. CoSA acknowledges this literature and does not in any way aim to shame the individual for their past behaviour, but instead supports the Core Member and focuses on active responsibility-taking. Furthermore, volunteers are encouraged to discuss the power of stigmatising labels such as 'sex offender' and 'paedophile' with the Core Member, and in fact the simple use of the neutral term Core Member serves to remove the individual from their previous behaviour.

Another element of Braithwaite's theory of reintegrative shaming relates to the power of 'significant others' in deterring criminal behaviour. The idea is that shame associated with letting those close to us down and causing disapproval can serve to promote desistance. For individuals with sexual crime convictions however, they are often ostracised from family and society, and so the idea of significant others may be something alien to these individuals. However, when part of CoSA, research suggests that the volunteers become a very important and integral part of the Core Member's life and social circle, and Braithwaite's role of significant others can be seen at play. For example, a CoSA coordinator stated 'Sometimes I get the feeling that they [Core Members] are like children, and that we are their family and that they'd disappoint us if they reoffended. That's it, I think—they don't want to disappoint us' (Silverman & Wilson, 2002, p. 173). This relates back to the idea of inclusion referred to above, as it is the 'family-like' relationships accomplished through CoSA that help the Core Member to once again feel a part of the community (Hannem, 2011 p. 278). Through this, Core Members have the opportunity to demonstrate change in the community (Höing, Vogelvang, & Bogaerts, 2015) as they 'buy into a sense of doing good and not letting fellow group members down'. It is through this sense of belonging to the CoSA group that Core Members are reinforced to take responsibility for their behaviour and ultimately be accountable (Kewley, 2017).

CoSA and Social Capital

A large body of research has highlighted how individuals convicted of sexual crime are publicly denigrated in the extreme and consequently find it more difficult than other types of offenders to reintegrate (Levenson & Cotter, 2005; Braden et al., 2012). Research has also found that public shaming and the subsequent social isolation experienced by those convicted of sexual crime constitute risk factors in terms of further offending, and this has prompted the emergence of various reintegration initiatives (Braden et al., 2012). The paradox of further isolating released individuals with sexual crime convictions is that it increases their risk of further offending and like many offenders they find themselves 'in' but not 'of' society (Irwin & Owen, 2005). Recent research has found that the social resources people have, that is, their social capital can be a massive contributor to crime 'desistance'. Such resources/capital are linked to protective factors. Social capital has been defined as "a network of relationships, which facilitates social action by generating knowledge and a sense of obligation, expectation, and trust" (Göbbels et al., 2012, p. 456).

Ullrich and Coid (2011) examined the predictors of desistance in 800 sexual and violent offenders. The only four significant protective factors were all related to pro-social supportive networks: social support, emotional support, spare time spent with family and friends, and closeness to others. Farmer et al. (2012) found that a main distinguishing feature between active and desisting individuals with sexual crime convictions was that the latter had found a place within a social group or network. Thus, having support, belonging to a group and being believed in cannot be under estimated in the desistance process (Maruna, 2001). CoSA can assist in this process and be a social resource which provides support and inclusion, while holding the individual to account (Höing et al., 2013). The process of being in a Circle, and being supported by those in the community, provides a 'surrogate social network', which assists the Core Member in developing their own personal social networks that are appropriate and pro-social (Höing et al., 2013, p. 271). This process is important as it has been found that forming new and meaningful relationships can provide individuals with the emotional and social capital they need to sustain a crime free life (Farmer et al., 2016).

Narratives of Re-entry and CoSA

There are three narratives of re-entry described by Maruna and LeBel (2002): control, support, and strength based. Control narratives are risk-based and are embedded within a belief that those who have committed crimes are dangerous and must be monitored and controlled at all times (Maruna & LeBel, 2002). In the UK, this is the basis of most interventions with those who have committed sexual crime in the community. The focus is heavily on supervision and management of risk through organisations such as MAPPA (Multi-Agency Public Protection Arrangements) and MOSOVO (Management of Sexual Offenders and Violent Offenders).

Support based narratives are arguably the direct opposite of control narratives. The idea here is to provide support and care based on individual needs, specifically and most importantly, their criminogenic needs (Maruna & LeBel, 2002). This concept is supported by the literature regarding 'What Works', which attempts to demonstrate that treatment can effectively reduce recidivism when an individual's criminogenic needs are directly matched to treatment. However, this approach is focused on *doing to* the ex-prisoners, through for example treatment in the community. As was mentioned earlier in this chapter, working with offenders rather than *on them* is crucial to the desistance process. Without this, individuals are not discovering agency or owning their rehabilitation.

This leads into an alternative and emerging narrative, titled 'strength based'. The idea behind this narrative is to build on the existing capabilities and capacities of individuals to support change. The concept is about looking at the strengths of individuals and identifying what positive contributions they are able to make. This is in complete contrast to the control narrative which focuses on deficits and areas of need. This is arguably the narrative within which CoSA sits most comfortably. Although it should be noted that CoSA runs the risk of acting as another social control, along with supervision and the other community requirements that are made on ex-prisoners. This is due to the 'accountability' element of CoSA, which should be adopted appropriately and with caution, or it may undermine the other strength based components of CoSA which arguably have the greatest potential in terms of desistance (McNeill, 2014). CoSA's focus on community integration by use of community volunteers heavily supports the resocialisation of Core Members and works to counteract some of the negative consequences of imprisonment.

This narrative links in with the Good Lives Model (GLM: e.g. Ward, 2002a, 2002b; Ward & Stewart, 2003), which provides a strength based approach to rehabilitation and desistance. The central premise of the GLM is that there are a number of 'actions, states of affairs, characteristics, experiences and states of mind that are intrinsically beneficial to human beings and therefore sought for their own sake' (Ward & Brown, 2004, p. 246). These are defined by the GLM as primary human goods. Specifically, eleven primary goods have been identified: life; knowledge; excellence in work; excellence in play; excellence in agency; inner peace; relatedness; community; spirituality; pleasure; and creativity (Purvis, 2010). According to the GLM, offending is the result of attempting to pursue primary goods through inappropriate methods. As such, from this perspective the rehabilitation of offenders focuses on providing opportunities, building capabilities and supporting individuals to achieve these via appropriate means in order to reduce the risk of reoffending and allow individuals to live fulfilling, crime free lives. CoSA are well aligned to the GLM, in that it aims to support Core Members in achieving human goods via pro-social methods in order to construct a balanced, fulfilled and socially supported crime free life (Bates, Macrae, Williams & Webb, 2012; Wilson, Cortoni, & McWhinnie, 2009). CoSA goes beyond the focus of criminogenic needs and targeted risk reduction and instead looks at individual needs, something that traditional programmes often fail to fully address due to practical barriers (Wilson & Yates, 2009). CoSA offers 'goods' such as support, advice and human communication which in turn increase wellbeing, enabling individuals to meet their needs in a prosocial way rather than through crime.

Conclusion

It is clear that the current predilection for exclusionary "criminology of the other" (Garland, 2001) type attitudes particularly focused at individuals with sexual crime convictions will not serve our communities' best interests. However, rehabilitative initiatives like CoSA and the simple acts associated with community inclusion and de-labelling of offenders promote enhanced (normative) identities among ex-offenders (Fox, 2015). They also provide a greater sense of sense of empowerment, autonomy, and contribution to a positive culture (Arrigo & Takahashi, 2006). This chapter has demonstrated how CoSA fits with the desistance literature and how they can contribute to the developing of a positive narrative and identity of the self and to improve human and social capital.

References

Arrigo, B. A., & Takahashi, Y. (2006). Recommunalization of the disenfranchised: A theoretical and critical criminological inquiry. *Theoretical Criminology, 10*(3), 307–336.

Bates, A., Macrae, R., Williams, D., & Webb, C. (2012). Ever-increasing circles: A descriptive study of Hampshire and Thames Valley circles of support and accountability 2002–09. *Journal of Sexual Aggression, 18*(3), 355–373.

Blagden, N., & Perrin, C. (2016). 'Relax lads, you're in safe hands here': Experiences of a sexual offender treatment prison. In C. Reeves (Ed.), *Experiencing prison* (pp. 27–45). Routledge.

Blagden, N., Perrin, C., Smith, S., Gleeson, F., & Gillies, L. (2017). "A different world" exploring and understanding the climate of a recently re-rolled sexual offender prison. *Journal of Sexual Aggression*. https://doi.org/10.1080/13552600.2016.1264633

Blagden, N., Winder, B., & Hames, C. (2014). "They treat us like human beings"—Experiencing a therapeutic sex offenders prison impact on prisoners and staff and implications for treatment. *International Journal of Offender Therapy and Comparative Criminology, 60*, 371–396. https://doi.org/10.1177/0306624X14553227

Blagden, N. J., Winder, B., Thorne, K., & Gregson, M. (2011). 'No-one in the world would ever wanna speak to me again': An interpretative phenomenological analysis into convicted sexual offenders accounts and experiences of maintaining and leaving denial. *Psychology, Crime & Law, 17*(7), 563–585.

Braden, M., Göbbels, S., Willis, G. M., Ward, T., Costeletos, M., & Mollica, J. (2012). Creating social capital and reducing harm: Corrections Victoria support and awareness groups. *Sexual Abuse in Australia and New Zealand, 4*(2), 36.

Braithwaite, J. (1989). *Crime, shame and reintegration*. Cambridge, UK: Cambridge University Press.
Brown, S. (1999). Public attitudes toward the treatment of sex offenders. *Legal and Criminological Psychology, 4*(2), 239–252.
Burnett, R., & McNeill, F. (2005). The place of the officer-offender relationship in assisting offenders to desist from crime. *Probation Journal, 52*(3), 221–242.
Cesaroni, C. (2001). Releasing sex offenders into the community through "circles of support"—A means of reintegrating the "worst of the worst". *Journal of Offender Rehabilitation, 34*(2), 85–98.
Chiricos, T., Barrick, K., & Bales, W. (2007). The labelling of convicted felons and its consequences for recidivism. *Criminology, 45*(3), 547–581.
Craig, L. A. (2005). The impact of training on attitudes towards sex offenders. *Journal of Sexual Aggression, 11*(2), 197–207.
de Vries Robbé, M., Mann, R. E., Maruna, S., & Thornton, D. (2015). An exploration of protective factors supporting desistance from sexual offending. *Sexual Abuse: A Journal of Research and Treatment, 27*(1), 16–33.
Elliott, I. A., & Zajac, G. (2015). The implementation of circles of support and accountability in the United States. *Aggression and Violent Behavior, 25*, 113–123.
Farmer, M., Beech, A. R., & Ward, T. (2012). Assessing desistance in child molesters: A qualitative analysis. *Journal of interpersonal Violence, 27*(5), 930–950.
Farmer, M., McAlinden, A. M., & Maruna, S. (2016). Sex offending and situational motivation: Findings from a qualitative analysis of desistance from sexual offending. *International Journal of Offender Therapy and Comparative Criminology, 60*(15), 1756–1775.
Fox, K. J. (2015). Theorizing community integration as desistance-promotion. *Criminal Justice and Behavior, 42*(1), 82–94.
Friestad, C. (2012). Making sense, making good, or making meaning? Cognitive distortions as targets of change in offender treatment. *International Journal of Offender Therapy and Comparative Criminology, 56*(3), 465–482.
Garland, D. (2001). *The culture of control* (Vol. 367). Oxford: Oxford University Press.
Göbbels, S., Ward, T., & Willis, G. M. (2012). An integrative theory of desistance from sex offending. *Aggression and Violent Behaviour, 17*(5), 453–462.
Hannem, S. (2011). Experiences in reconciling risk management and restorative justice: How circles of support and accountability work restoratively in the risk society. *International Journal of Offender Therapy and Comparative Criminology, 57*(3), 269–288.

Höing, M., Bogaerts, S., & Vogelvang, B. (2013). Circles of support and accountability: How and why they work for sex offenders. *Journal of Forensic Psychology Practice, 13*(4), 267–295.
Höing, M., Vogelvang, B., & Bogaerts, S. (2015). "I am a different man now"—Sex offenders in circles of support and accountability: A prospective study. *International Journal of Offender Therapy and Comparative Criminology, 61*(7), 751–722.
Horvath, A. O., & Greenberg, L. S. (1989). Development and validation of the working alliance inventory. *Journal of Counseling Psychology, 36*(2), 223–233. https://doi.org/10.1037/0022-0167.36.2.223
Horvath, A. O., & Luborsky, L. (1993). The role of the therapeutic alliance in psychotherapy. *Journal of Consulting and Clinical Psychology, 61*(4), 561–573. https://doi.org/10.1037/0022-006X.61.4.561
Irwin, J., & Owen, B. (2005). Harm and the contemporary prison. In A. Liebling & S. Maruna (Eds.), *The effects of imprisonment* (pp. 94–117). London: Willan.
Kewley, S. (2017). Strength based approaches and protective factors from a criminological perspective. *Aggression and Violent Behavior, 32*, 11–18.
Kitson-Boyce, R., Blagden, N., Winder, B., & Dillon, G. (2016). The CoSA prison-model: Supporting the transition from prison to community. In *16th Annual Conference of the European Society of Criminology 2016*, University of Münster, Münster, Germany, 21–24 September.
Kjelsberg, E., & Loos, L. H. (2008). Conciliation or condemnation? Prison employees' and young peoples' attitudes towards sexual offender. *International Journal of Forensic Mental Health, 7*(1), 95–103.
LeBel, T. P., Burnett, R., Maruna, S., & Bushway, S. (2008). The chicken and egg'of subjective and social factors in desistance from crime. *European Journal of Criminology, 5*(2), 131–159.
Levenson, J. S., & Cotter, L. P. (2005). The effect of Megan's Law on sex offender reintegration. *Journal of Contemporary Criminal Justice, 21*(1), 49–66.
Maruna, S. (2001). *Making good: How ex-convicts reform and rebuild their lives.* Washington, DC: American Psychological Association.
Maruna, S. (2004). Desistance from crime and explanatory style: A new direction in the psychology of reform. *Journal of Contemporary Criminal Justice, 20*(2), 184–200.
Maruna, S., & LeBel, T. P. (2002). Welcome home? Examining the "reentry court" concept from a strengths-based perspective. *Western Criminology Review, 4*, 91.

Maruna, S., LeBel, T., Naples, M., & Mitchell, N. (2009). Looking-glass identity transformation: Pygmalion and Golem in the rehabilitation process. In *How offenders transform their lives* (pp. 30–55). Cullompton, UK: Willan.

McAdams, D. P. (2006a). The redemptive self: Generativity and the stories Americans live by. *Research in Human Development, 3*(2–3), 81–100.

McAdams, D. P. (2006b). The role of narrative in personality psychology today. *Narrative Inquiry, 16*(1), 11–18.

McAlinden, A. M. (2007). *The shaming of individuals with sexual crime convictions: Risk, retribution and reintegration.* Bloomsbury Publishing.

McCulloch, T. (2005). Probation, social context and desistance: Retracing the relationship. *Probation Journal, 52*(1), 8–22.

McNeill, F. (2014, May). Desistance, rehabilitation and reintegration. In J. Shapland (Chair), *How best to stop offenders re-offending and reintegrate them into civil society.* Symposium conducted at the seminar series of the University of Sheffield Centre for Criminological Research, London, UK.

Mead, S., Hilton, D., & Curtis, L. (2001). Peer support: A theoretical perspective. *Psychiatric Rehabilitation Journal, 25*(2), 134.

Paternoster, R., & Bushway, S. (2009). Desistance and the "feared self": Toward an identity theory of criminal desistance. *The Journal of Criminal Law and Criminology, 99,* 1103–1156.

Perrin, C., & Blagden, N. (2014). Accumulating meaning, purpose and opportunities to change 'drip by drip': The impact of being a listener in prison. *Psychology, Crime & Law, 20*(9), 902–920.

Petrunik, M. (2003). The hare and the tortoise: Dangerousness and sex offender policy in the United States and Canada. *Canadian Journal of Criminology and Criminal Justice, 45,* 43–72.

Purvis, M. (2010). *Seeking a good life: Human goods and sexual offending.* Germany: Lambert Academic Press.

Rogers, C. R. (1951). *Client-centered therapy.* Boston: Houghton Mifflin.

Silverman, J., & Wilson, D. (2002). *Innocence betrayed: Paedophilia, the media and society.* Cambridge, UK: Polity.

Stone, R. (2015). Desistance and identity repair: Redemption narratives as resistance to stigma. *British Journal of Criminology.* https://doi.org/10.1093/BJC/AZV081

Tate, H., Blagden, N., & Mann, R. (in press). *Evaluation the five minute intervention.* London: MoJ.

Ullrich, S., & Coid, J. (2011). Protective factors for violence among released prisoners—Effects over time and interactions with static risk. *Journal of Consulting and Clinical psychology, 79*(3), 381.

Vaughan, B. (2007). The internal narrative of desistance. *British Journal of Criminology, 47*(3), 390–404.
Ward, T. (2002a). Good lives and the rehabilitation of offenders: Promises and problems. *Aggression and Violent Behavior, 7*(5), 513–528.
Ward, T. (2002b). The management of risk and the design of good lives. *Australian Psychologist, 37*, 172–179.
Ward, T., & Brown, M. (2004). The good lives model and conceptual issues in offender rehabilitation. *Psychology, Crime, & Law, 10*, 243–257.
Ward, T., & Marshall, B. (2007). Narrative identity and offender rehabilitation. *International Journal of Offender Therapy and Comparative Criminology, 51*(3), 279–297.
Ward, T., & Stewart, C. A. (2003). The treatment of sex offenders: Risk management and good lives. *Professional Psychology: Research and Practice, 34*, 353–360.
Weaver, B. (2015). *Offending and desistance: The importance of social relations* (Vol. 8). London: Routledge.
Weaver, B., & McNeill, F. (2015). Lifelines: Desistance, social relations, and reciprocity. *Criminal Justice and Behavior, 42*(1), 95–107.
Wilson, R. J., Cortoni, F., & McWhinnie, A. J. (2009). Circles of support & accountability: A Canadian national replication of outcome findings. *Sexual Abuse, 21*(4), 412–430.
Wilson, R. J., & Yates, P. M. (2009). Effective interventions and the Good Lives Model: Maximizing treatment gains for individuals with sexual crime convictions. *Aggression and Violent Behavior, 14*(3), 157–161.
Youssef, C., Casey, S., & Birgden, A. (2017). Potential underpinnings for community maintenance programs for individuals with sexual crime convictions. *Aggression and Violent Behavior*. https://doi.org/10.1016/j.avb.2017.05.002

3

Do Circles of Support and Accountability Work? A Review of the Literature

Rosie Kitson-Boyce

To ensure that CoSA projects continue to grow in both success and public confidence on an international scale, a solid research base is essential. In addition, to inform best practice the factors involved in the success of CoSA need to be identified (Wilson, Bates, & Völlm, 2010). The following chapter focuses upon the growing body of efficacy research surrounding CoSA projects. This will include the key statistical evaluations of the effect of CoSA on recidivism, along with more qualitative explorations of the psychosocial implications of being involved.

Do CoSA Reduce Recidivism?

In 2005, Wilson, Picheca and Prinzo carried out the first evaluation of the CoSA pilot project in South-Central Ontario, Canada. The evaluation was split into two parts, with the second part (Wilson et al., 2005; Wilson, Picheca, & Prinzo, 2007b) assessing specifically the rates of

R. Kitson-Boyce (✉)
Nottingham Trent University, Nottingham, UK

H. Elliott et al. (eds.), *Sexual Crime and Circles of Support and Accountability*, Sexual Crime, https://doi.org/10.1007/978-3-319-74823-8_3

reoffending of those involved in CoSA compared to a matched sample of those who were not.

The reoffending comparison study consisted of two groups of offenders and an average follow up time of 4.5 years. The CoSA group consisted of 60 individuals previously convicted of a sexual crime, who had become involved in the CoSA project at the end of their sentence. The comparison sample involved 60 individuals also convicted of a sexual crime, who were released following completion of their prison sentence, but who did not participate in a CoSA. In order to eliminate potential confounding variables influencing the findings, Wilson et al. (2005, 2007b) endeavoured to match the groups on release date, risk category (e.g. low, moderate, moderate-high, high) and prior involvement in sex offender treatment programmes. However, the CoSA group had a significantly higher risk of sexual recidivism than the comparison group (assessed using the RRASOR; Rapid Risk Assessment for Sexual Offence Recidivism; Hanson, 1997), and a significantly higher average of number of victims. This resulted in a comparison group who would presumably therefore reoffend at a lower rate than the CoSA group. As the authors acknowledged, in order for the matching process to be exact, the two groups should not have differed in this way, with regard to risk. The deficiencies in the matching protocol of the two groups were argued to be a consequence of the resource difficulties the CoSA project faced. The limited services resulted in a selection bias whereby CoSA were allocated to those individuals most in need, that is at the highest risk of reoffending.

Despite the higher risk profile of the CoSA group, however, the comparison group reoffended at a faster and higher rate than the CoSA group. It was reported that being a Core Member of CoSA resulted in a reduction in sexual recidivism when compared to individuals who were not in CoSA (5% sexual recidivism in the CoSA group vs. 16.7% sexual recidivism in the comparison group), demonstrating that the comparison group reoffended at three times the rate of the CoSA group. There was also a 57% reduction in all types of violent recidivism; 15% violent (and sexual) recidivism in the CoSA group vs. 35% violent (and sexual) recidivism in the comparison group. Overall there was a reduction of 35% in all types of recidivism; 28.3% in the CoSA group vs. 43.4% in the comparison group. Alongside this, the three instances of sexual reoffending in the CoSA group were described by Wilson et al. (2007b, p. 332) to be 'qualitatively less severe or invasive than the offence for which they had most recently served sentence'. Details were only given however, for one out of the three instances, whereby a Core Member, whose previous conviction was for rape, reoffended by making an obscene phone call. This shift from perpetration of a contact offence, to a non-contact offence is described within the literature as a harm reduction function of CoSA and therefore still viewed as a positive and encouraging finding (Wilson et al., 2005, 2007b, 2010). However, it is unknown as to whether this reduction in harm occurred for all three reoffences.

As CoSA projects spread throughout Canada, Wilson, Cortoni, and McWhinnie (2009) sought to replicate the findings of the pilot study evaluation (Wilson et al., 2005, 2007b), by examining whether CoSA continued to demonstrate efficacy in reducing recidivism. Using a similar methodology, 44 offenders, previously convicted for a sexual crime and who were involved in CoSA, were matched on general risk, time of and geographical location of release and prior participation in sex offender treatment programmes, to a comparison sample of 44 offenders who were not involved in CoSA. It is important to note here that in all cases of CoSA research, the voluntary nature of participating in CoSA may result in a self-selection bias. For example, CoSA may be found to be successful in reducing recidivism due to the Core Members already having made the decision to leave their life of crime behind. This cannot be proven however, due to authors such as Farrall (2002) arguing that early aspirations and motivations to change do not guarantee that desistance from crime will take place.

The risk between the CoSA and comparison group was determined, using the risk assessment tool STATIC-99 (Hanson & Thornton, 2000) and like the previous study, a statistically significant difference was reported. In the case of these two samples however, it was the comparison group who produced the higher average risk scores. Similar to the previous study though, the results demonstrated that the reoffending rates for those in the CoSA group were significantly lower than for those in the comparison group. Specifically, when comparing the CoSA group to the matched comparison group, there was an 83% reduction in sexual recidivism (2.3% CoSA vs. 13.7% Comparison), a 73% reduction in all types

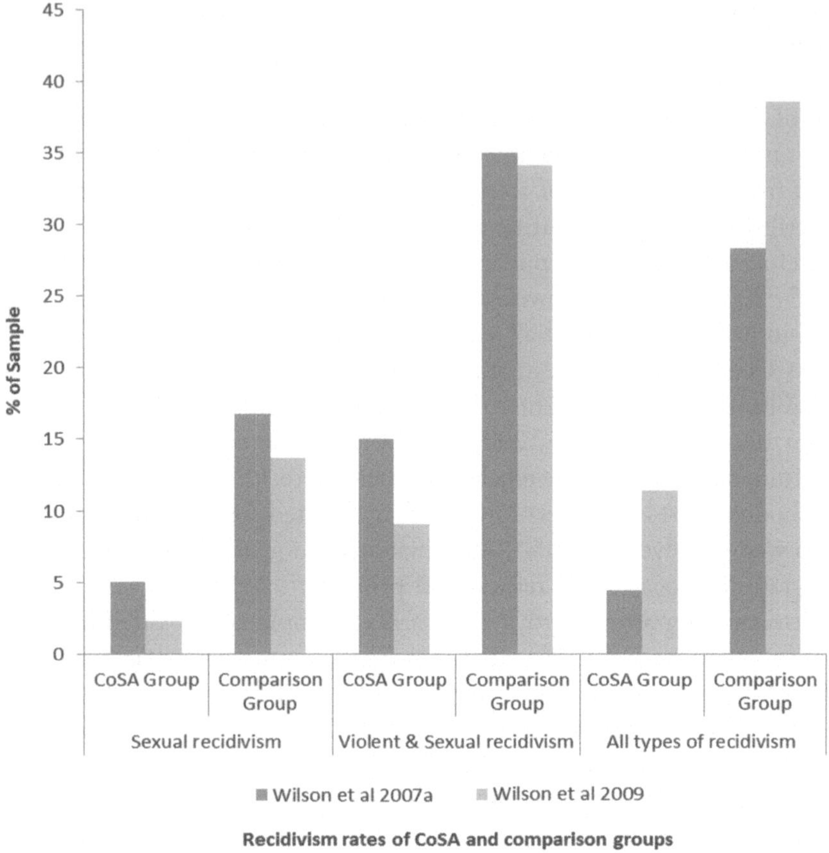

Fig. 3.1 Recidivism rates taken from Wilson et al. (2007a, 2009)

of violent recidivism (9.1% CoSA vs. 34.1% Comparison) and a 70% overall reduction in all types of recidivism (11.4% CoSA vs. 38.6% Comparison). The differences in recidivism rates are comparable to the previous study outlined, as can be seen in the figure below (Fig. 3.1).

Despite using a shorter follow up period (3 years) than the 2005 study, Wilson et al. (2010) argue that the latter research supports the findings that CoSA are an effective rehabilitative and restorative initiative for high risk offenders who commit sexual offences. It is acknowledged however, that the lesser risk profile in the CoSA group, compared to the matched offenders weakens the robustness of the findings (Wilson et al., 2009). In addition to this, Elliott, Zajac, and Meyer (2013) argued that if a Fisher's Exact Test had been used to analyse the results instead of the chi-square distribution test, as would be recommended due to the small number of recidivists, then a non-significant result would have been reported.

Alongside the above, Canadian research into CoSA has been criticised for providing limited information about the methods that were used to identify a suitable comparison group, and for basing their studies on small sample sizes (McCartan, Kemshall, Westwood, MacKenzie, & Pollard, 2014). Elliot and Zajac (2015) also make this argument, stating that in both studies, details of the methods used to match the groups for prior treatment was not described nor do the researchers explain why the control sample did not participate in CoSA. If the reason was that they were not suitable to participate, they may not have represented an adequate control sample due to confounding differences with the experimental group.

UK CoSA

Following the establishment of the CoSA pilot projects in the UK (for a detailed history of CoSA in the UK see Chap. 1), an evaluation of the first four years of the Thames Valley CoSA project was carried out by Bates, Saunders, and Wilson (2007). Different to the efficacy studies carried out in Canada, case files of the Core Members registered with CoSA between November 2002 and May 2006 (n = 16) were reviewed in the study. Although, as the authors acknowledged, the follow-up period (less than 4 years) was inadequate for a formal reconviction study, none of the Core Members involved in the CoSA reviewed were reconvicted of a sexual offence. This suggested that, as in the studies from other countries, involvement in CoSA may have reduced the likelihood of reoffending.

A detailed analysis found that one Core Member (6.3%) was convicted of a breach of a Sex Offence Prevention Order, four (25%) were recalled for breaching the conditions of their parole licence and five (31.3%) were reported to exhibit some form of recidivist behaviour. These outcomes, however, were still deemed as a success due to the fact that early intervention was possible and no further victims were created (Wilson, McWhinnie, & Wilson, 2008). The authors went on to argue that breaches of parole and return to prison should not necessarily be regarded as a 'failure' due to the role that CoSA and the volunteers had played in gathering intelligence and passing this on, resulting in the prevention of further sexual abuse. Further to this, of the four recalled to prison, three retained contact with CoSA and returned as a Core Member for ongoing support on release. As Wilson et al. (2010) acknowledge, this provides clear evidence of the ability for the support and accountability elements of CoSA to co-exist alongside one another.

Another explanation for the results is that additional contact with ex-offenders through CoSA may inflate the detection of new offences (Elliott & Beech, 2012), meaning offence-related behaviour is being reported that would otherwise go undetected. Although CoSA in the UK has risk management alongside successful offender reintegration as its joint focus, it is argued that its ability to address recidivism is the sole attraction for support and funding of the initiative (Hannem & Petrunik, 2007). Some even go as far as to argue that initiatives such as CoSA are actually just a widening of the net of formal social control, under a disguise of reintegration or restoration (Hannem, 2011), a view that is contested by CoSA providers in the UK.

In 2012, Bates, Macrae, Williams and Webb were able to expand upon the above findings, focusing on the first 8 years of CoSA within the UK. Case files for the sample (n = 60) included information about each Core Member, since the beginning of their involvement with CoSA and during the follow-up period since. This included descriptive demographic information and outcome data (e.g. recall, reconviction, successful reintegration), which was examined and evaluated. These methods have been criticised however, due to a lack of objective measurement and an over-reliance on the researcher's judgement of the file information, making it difficult to ascertain whether the improvements reported were in fact due to taking part in CoSA (Elliott et al., 2013).

Nevertheless, 75% of the CoSA analysed were categorised as having a positive outcome, with any problematic behaviours demonstrated by the Core Members managed within the CoSA itself. Of the 25% deemed to have not completed successfully, two Core Members had demonstrated behaviour that paralleled previous offending behaviour, resulting in Sex Offence Prevention Orders being made. Alongside this, one Core Member (1.6%) was reconvicted of a sexual offence and sentenced to 15 months imprisonment for downloading images of sexual abuse. Since the sexual reconviction was for an internet offence, as opposed to contact offending, the CoSA was still reported as making positive progress by the authors, through reducing the Core Member's risk of harm and the severity of his offending behaviour.

Although the studies discussed here go some way to demonstrating the efficacy of CoSA, they have been criticised for the use of small sample sizes (Wilson & McWhinnie, 2013). Armstrong and Wills (2014b) explain how the lack of any large-scale research of reoffending post CoSA is attributable to the low base rate for sexual offending in the first place. For example, Hanson and Morton-Bourgon (2009) recently reported a sexual recidivism rate of 11.5%, which is comparatively low when comparing to recidivism rates for any new offence (33.2%). In addition, projects within the UK specifically face criticism due to the absence of a comparison group (Duwe, 2012). Bates et al. (2012) acknowledged this limitation to their research, which Hanvey, Philpot, and Wilson (2011) agreed with by stating that a comparison group matched to Core Members on as many variables as possible, in relation to the prediction of reoffending, is an ideal method to be used in CoSA efficacy studies.

In an attempt to overcome these criticisms Bates, Williams, Wilson, and Wilson (2014) carried out a larger comparison study on 71 of the 100 CoSA established in the South East of the UK since its commencement. Unlike previous efficacy studies of CoSA, this research involved a ten-year follow up period, which is considered by some to be a credible length from which to derive conclusions of effectiveness (Hanvey et al., 2011). The average time a Core Member was involved in CoSA was 15.9 months, with the average follow up period being four years and four months. Behavioural outcomes of the Core Members, along with formal reconviction data were reviewed and compared to a group of 71 offenders, convicted of sexual offences who were referred to, but did not receive CoSA. Reasons for not receiving CoSA were lack of availability, lack of motivation to engage or withdrawal after being assessed as suitable. Although both groups were matched as having broadly similar risk scores using the RM2000 risk assessment tool (Thornton et al., 2003) and therefore held similar projection rates of reoffending, the Core Members actually reoffended sexually or violently at a lower rate than those who were not involved with CoSA.

Out of the 71 Core Members involved in CoSA, 54 had not engaged in any criminal behaviour involving a legal sanction, since formally starting their CoSA. Of the 17 Core Members that did, three were identified as having nonsexual reconvictions, four obtained convictions for failing to comply with the Sex Offender's Register requirements and another four returned to prison due to violating the terms of their conditional release. In addition, two Core Members were convicted for violating the terms of their Sex Offence Prevention Order (SOPO). In one of these cases, this was following the CoSA reporting the violation to the police. Similarly, one Core Member was subject to a SOPO during his time on CoSA due to concerns about his behaviour. This arguably still demonstrates CoSA's effectiveness, due to action being taken before any future victims were created. Finally, four sexual reconvictions were identified within the Core Members, one for a historical sexual offence and three for non-contact sexual offences. For two of the non-contact offences, previous offences had been for a contact sexual offence, therefore, similar to previous efficacy studies, a harm reduction effect was documented by the authors when compared to their original conviction.

Despite the above, in terms of actual versus expected re-offences (using the risk levels of the RM2000 tool), neither group reoffended sexually at a rate significantly different to that which was predicted (Elliott, 2014; Elliott & Zajac, 2015). In addition, Bates et al. (2014) included a '90 day rule' to the sample in their study, in order to ensure Core Members had sufficient time to have benefited from the CoSA process. The rule stipulated that only Core Members who had been with CoSA for a minimum of 90 days would be included in the study. This was based on the assumption that those who had spent less than 90 days in their CoSA would not have not have had sufficient time to have significantly benefited from their involvement.

Their rationale for the inclusion of this was stated as being due to the use of such a rule in prior Canadian studies. However, as Elliott and Zajac (2015) highlight, no reference of this is made in either of the Canadian studies that have been outlined earlier in this chapter. If such an exclusion criteria was used then one could question the extent to which the true effectiveness of CoSA are reported. This is due to the early stages of release from prison, being a particularly sensitive period in terms of desistance (Aresti, Eatough, & Brooks-Gordon, 2010), with reoffending expected to occur within the first few weeks (Elliott & Zajac, 2015). Indeed, the authors themselves reported how, during this 90 day period, five Core Members had been recalled to prison for breach of licence conditions and four withdrew from their CoSA; all of which were excluded under the 90 day rule. The use of a 90 day rule in CoSA efficacy research, such as Bates et al. (2014), therefore excludes data from a period during which there is a higher likelihood of CoSA failures and Core Member dropouts (Elliott & Zajac, 2015).

In conclusion Bates et al. (2014) highlight how a Core Member's lack of ability to refrain from reoffending may not relate entirely to the quality (or lack thereof) of support and accountability (Bates et al., 2014). Instead an individual's motivation to desist from offending or the opportunities available to them to access a balanced, self-determined lifestyle consistent with the theories outlined in Chap. 2 also need to be considered. In addition, although the length of follow-up and the use of a reasonable comparison group were comparable to the CoSA efficacy studies carried out in Canada, Bates et al. (2014) acknowledge that using a randomised clinical trial, or matched participants, would have been preferable.

The RCT Debate

The only study to date that has randomly assigned participants to either an experimental group (CoSA) or a control group (non-CoSA), was carried out by Duwe (2012) in the US. Duwe (2012) utilised a Randomised Control Trial (RCT) design by randomly assigning 62 men, previously convicted of sexual offences, to either an experimental group, whereby they took part in CoSA, or a control group, where they did not. All of the participants involved in the study had previously been deemed suitable for the Minnesota CoSA programme and expressed interest in becoming involved, therefore controlling for offender motivation. As Elliott, Zajac, and Meyer (2013) point out, using this randomised procedure goes some way to resolving the issue of potential differences between CoSA and a control group. The findings of the study were not however as positive as the previous mentioned results. There were no significant reductions in the reconviction or re-incarceration rates. However, a statistically significant reduction in re-arrest for any offence (38.7% CMs vs 64.5% controls) was reported, as well as a non-significant reduction in sexual recidivism over a 2 year follow up (0% CMs vs 3.2% control). The short follow up period of the study was held responsible for the lack of a statistically significant results (Wilson & McWhinnie, 2013).

The use of short follow up periods is a limitation consistent across CoSA research internationally (McCartan et al., 2014; Thomas, Thompson, & Karstedt, 2014; Wilson & McWhinnie, 2013). Cann, Falshaw, and Friendship (2004) reported from a reconviction study involving a 21 year follow up period, that individuals convicted previously for sexual offences, were actually at risk of reoffending for many years after being released from prison. The sample consisted of 413 participants previously convicted of a sexual crime, 103 of whom reoffended sexually during the 21 years they were followed. Thus, using a 5-year follow up period, with the same individuals, may have missed over one third (36%) of new sexual re-offences, with one fifth of those who reoffended living offence-free lives for at least ten years before committing their first sexual re-offence. Although there are many limitations of using such a long follow up period, that is the research can become out-dated by the time of publication, it does provide evidence of individuals who have remained offence free for many years (see Cann et al., 2004 for more detail). This demonstrates that using a short follow up period similar to that of the CoSA research will not always provide an accurate picture of the true impact of CoSA on reconviction rates.

With regard to study design, the use of RCTs is often considered the 'gold standard' in evaluation research. However, it is not always a straightforward process when applying this design to those who commit sexual offences. With regard to sex offender treatment Marques, Wiederanders, Day, Nelson, and van Ommeren (2005) conducted an RCT which uncovered some significant design issues, one in particular which is relevant to the use of an RCT in CoSA research. Participants in the treatment group all received exactly the same number of treatment sessions over the same length of time, in line with the requirements of an RCT design. No treatment effect was found within the study, possibly due to the fact that the treatment had been developed to be tailored to each individual and their needs, in order to be effective (Marshall & Marshall, 2007). Indeed, desistance is both an individualised and subjective process (McNeill, 2009) meaning that one-size-fits-all interventions will not always work. CoSA therefore, works with the Core Member on an individual basis and offers support that is specific to their needs. A strict RCT design may change the length and content of the CoSA sessions, reducing the individualised nature and therefore undermining the potential effectiveness.

In addition to design issues, Marshall and Marshall (2007) argue that RCTs are unethical, when used with individuals who have committed sexual offences, due to the control group being denied access to a programme or treatment. In the case of CoSA, whereby those participating are at a high risk of reoffending sexually and are due for release in to the community, the use of RCTs becomes an ethically questionable concept (Lussier & Gress, 2014). Hanvey et al. (2011) highlight the ethical issues surrounding the use of RCTs to demonstrate CoSA effectiveness, stating that the use of a control group denies individuals at risk of committing further sexual crime a place on a supportive initiative that has already been shown to reduce risk of reoffending. Duwe (2012) countered this criticism of his study however, by explaining that the use of an RCT design did not result in any individual being denied involvement in CoSA purely for the benefit of the research. Instead, he stated, that the number of individuals, willing and able to take part in CoSA, exceeded the number of volunteers and therefore CoSA available. One could still question however, whether it is ethical to engage in discussions with individuals regarding motivation and willingness to engage in CoSA, in the knowledge that places will not be available for everyone.

In summary, despite a growing body of literature regarding CoSA efficacy, critics have argued that there is not yet enough evidence to suggest whether or not CoSA significantly reduces sexual recidivism by the Core Member, with existing research varying in quality and involving a lack of statistically significant results (Elliott et al., 2013). In part, due to some of these limitations of the quantitative data, calls have been made for further qualitative evaluations in order to explore the factors contributing to the success of CoSA at a deeper level (McWhinnie, 2015). These will now be discussed in the following sections.

How Effective Are CoSA in Preventing Social Isolation?

In addition to considering the impact on recidivism rates, Wilson et al. (2007a), explored Core Members' experiences of being involved in CoSA and their motivations for participating. In line with the criteria for being selected as a Core Member, 83% of the participants reported that having no other form of social support was the main reason for deciding to take part in CoSA. Using a different sample to the recidivism study, over half of the twenty-four male offenders who had been convicted of a sexual offence, and were current or past Core Members, stated that negative community reaction to their release was also a motivating factor for becoming involved in CoSA. Worryingly, the study demonstrated the difficulties the Core Members would have had in adjusting to the community without being involved in CoSA, with the majority stating they would have felt lonely, isolated and powerless. This is particularly concerning given that isolation and emotional loneliness are significant risk factors in sexual recidivist behaviours (Hanson & Morton-Bourgon, 2005; Marshall, 2010) and indeed approximately two-thirds of the participants reported they thought they would have returned to crime without CoSA.

Being involved with the CoSA however, helped to combat this social isolation and loneliness with 92% of the Core Members stating they experienced a sense of support and acceptance when they first joined. They stated they would have tried anything to help them reintegrate back in society, and expressed relief and gratitude for having a Core Member place made available to them. These psychosocial outcomes are important to consider, due to a recognition within the literature that isolation and emotional loneliness can be factors significant in sexual recidivist behaviours (Hanson & Morton-Bourgon, 2005; Marshall, 2010). With its focus on support, however, CoSA provides a meaningful sense of belonging and inclusion, helping to counteract the social isolation and feelings of loneliness and rejection that are argued to be associated with sexual reoffending (Wilson et al., 2009).

Developing this body of research Fox (2015a) conducted the first qualitative study in the US, in order to explore the relationships formed between the Core Members and volunteers. Fox collected interview data from a sample that included both Core Members ($n = 20$) and volunteers ($n = 57$) from the CoSA project in Vermont, US. No established qualitative method was reported as being used to analyse the data, however details were given to suggest a form of thematic analysis was undertaken (Elliott & Zajac, 2015). It is also important to note that Vermont provides CoSA for individuals with a wider criminal history than just sexual offences, for example, high risk offenders, who have committed homicide (Fox, 2015b). All offence types were included in the research making it problematic when generalising the results to other CoSA projects who only include individuals convicted of at least one sexual offence.

From the results, Fox (2015a) reported how involvement in CoSA could help mitigate the isolation felt by many of the Core Members on their release from prison. In addition, they stated that CoSA created a space for the Core Members to practice and rehearse ordinary, pro-social relationships with members of the community and help support them in their ability to sustain pro-social healthy relationships. Although the Core Members reported motivation to desist from reoffending, they also explained how they felt excluded and labelled by the community due to their crimes. This is an issue that is very current in the literature, due to the barriers this ostracisation causes to successful reintegration (Mingus & Burchfield, 2012; Tewksbury, 2012). This is discussed at length within Chap. 6 of this book, where the media and societal views are explored. Fox (2015a) reported that the volunteers were combatting these feelings of exclusion through the inclusion of the Core Members. This created a sense of belonging for the Core Members, which Weaver and McNeill (2015) highlighted as being necessary for successful desistance from crime to take place. They reported from their research that social relations characterised this solidarity, supporting the individual to realise their aspirations, which in the case of CoSA, involved achieving a crime-free life, without feeling dependant. Following this, further research is now required to explore the context of the social bonds formed through CoSA, in relation specifically to the role they play in supporting the Core Member reach desistance from sexual offending (Fox, 2015a).

In summary, the qualitative nature of this research, particularly given the previous criticisms of the quantitative studies, helps to inform best practice, by identifying the factors involved in CoSA's success, something that Wilson et al. (2010) argue is critical. It is not without its criticisms, however, with the research outlined above involving small, unrepresentative samples. Nevertheless as Fox (2015a) argues, rather than determining the effect on recidivism, qualitative studies such as these provide an in-depth exploration in to a given topic, that is the impact CoSA has on reduction social isolation in those who commit sexual offences.

Can CoSA Improve Psychological Wellbeing?

Alongside research exploring the role of CoSA in the reduction of social isolation and loneliness, other psychosocial benefits, such as the impact of CoSA on Core Member's psychological wellbeing, are also considered within the literature. Bates, Macrae, Williams, and Webb's (2012) study sought to address the impact of CoSA on the life of a Core Member and the benefits of being involved. From their findings, it was reported that 70% resulted in an improvement in the Core Members' emotional wellbeing, due to their involvement with volunteers with whom they could relate and share issues with, thus reducing their emotional loneliness and social isolation. Nearly 50% of Core Members had improved links with their families, had increased their support networks, and were encouraged to access employment and education. Alongside this, 61% had displayed attitudes and behaviours that were pro-social and 50% had increased their engagement in age-appropriate relationships. This is of particular significance due to the fact that the majority of Core Members had been convicted previously of sexual crimes involving child victims (48/60).

Similarly in 2012, the Ministry of Justice commissioned a small independent study of the NOMS-funded CoSA pilot studies in order to understand the added support and value CoSA provides. Although no face-to-face data collection took place, file reviews of 32 Core Members revealed that the CoSA pilots had provided both practical and emotional support to the Core Members. In addition, the Core Members were able to successfully identify, develop and take part in prosocial activities and networks, such as safe leisure activities, volunteering, education courses and going to church (McCartan et al., 2014). Alongside this, 21/32 Core Members had been recorded as reporting positive changes in their motivations and attitudes after being involved with CoSA. These included increased coping skills, a reduction in anger, greater insight into offending and the development of coping strategies. Unlike previous studies, negative or mixed reports of CoSA were also documented. These included the Core Member having a lack of engagement, openness and honesty along with a reluctance to engage with the relapse prevention plan and manage their risk. Whilst it is essential to include all aspects of a CoSA project in order to make future improvements, the study did not document what the result of these negative cases were, for example whether the Core Member was recalled to prison or dropped out of the CoSA early (see Chap. 5 for more detail on this issue).

In 2013, Höing, Bogaerts, and Vogelvang (2013) conducted interviews with Core Members on Dutch (n = 10) and UK (n = 4) CoSA. A temporal card-sorting task (see Höing et al., 2013 for details on the exact procedure) was also administered in the Dutch CoSA with six of the Core Members, to further explore the categories and concepts derived from the interviews. Core Member progress was represented by less rumination and stress, more active problem solving behaviour and improved social and relationship skills. Some of the Core Members developed a more positive outlook on the future and their ability to live a 'normal' life. This finding in particular is significant due to the links made between hope and desistance. For example, LeBel, Burnett, Maruna, and Bushway

(2008) reported from their research with repeat offenders that a belief in one's ability to leave crime behind, along with a sense of hope, is a necessary condition for an individual to be able to desist from crime. Höing et al. (2013) also reported some of the difficulties faced by Core Members during their Circle, something that has been arguably missing from the early CoSA research generally (Elliott, 2014). Some of the Core Members had difficulties with open communication, especially at the beginning of their CoSA and the volunteer interviews in particular reported some Core Members' behaviour as secretive, avoidant and even manipulative.

From their findings, Höing et al. (2013) argued that in order to be effective in supporting the Core Member to successfully desist from sexual crime, CoSA must be inclusive; defined by trust, openness, belonging, equality and acceptance. These qualities support the internal motivation to change within the Core Member and provide a safe place for the new pro-social identity to be developed. Further evidence for this can be taken from Weaver and McNeill's (2015) research involving repeat offenders and the exploration of social relationships. They argued that it was the sense of belonging and social bonds, such as that Höing et al. (2013) highlighted within the CoSA they examined, that can encourage change within an individual and a shift towards desistance. In relation to the potential impact of social bonds being formed within CoSA, further research could consider how many of the Core Members displaying difficult communication behaviour or who withdraw from the process, are part of an inclusive CoSA. This would explore further the relationship between social bonds within the CoSA and it's 'success'.

To explore further the contribution of CoSA in the desistance process of the Core Members, Höing, Vogelvang and Bogaerts (2015) collected qualitative and quantitative data. Contrary to the other countries discussed so far, Core Members in this Netherlands CoSA project had to have completed, or currently be engaging in, a sex offender treatment programme (SOTP) before being accepted onto CoSA. Data collection took place at three different time points during the Core Members' CoSA journey and involved both interviews and questionnaires being administered (n = 17). The qualitative analysis discussed the internal and external transitions deemed to be necessary in order to reach successful desistance from crime (Paternoster & Bushway, 2009). After six months of being involved with CoSA, Core Members reported cognitive, internal transitions such as improvements in openness, self-reflection and assertiveness, along with the development of self-regulation and social skills. With regard to external transitions, little change was reported at the six month point, although two Core Members had begun to develop more appropriate leisure activities. In addition, some Core Members reported feelings of stress which they attributed to volunteers being too demanding or demonstrating excluding behaviour.

By the 12-month time point Höing, Vogelvang and Bogaerts (2015) reported a continuation of the positive changes in interpersonal skills, which they state coincided with increased self-confidence or a more positive self-image. Increased problem-solving skills were identified as the most prominent positive change from the Core Member interviews. External changes had also taken place by this point for some Core Members, with reports of improvements in existing relationships or the extension of social networks outside CoSA. Interestingly the quantitative data highlighted no improvement in the Core Members with regard to participation in society and the size of their own network. This leads to the question therefore, of how successful the CoSA had been, in terms of reintegrating the Core Member back in to the community and becoming a fully functioning member of society. In order to explore the impact of the low rate of external transitions reported by the Core Members, further research would be required over longer periods, which the authors highlight in their conclusions. Overall, the study demonstrates the positive impact being part of CoSA has for the Core Member with regard to making steps towards successful desistance.

In summary, the research appears to identify CoSA as having a positive impact on the psychological wellbeing of Core Members, resulting in substantial internal transitions towards a crime-free life. Although Core Members appear, through the support of the CoSA, to be progressing towards desistance, further research after the CoSA journey has ended, would help to determine whether this was in fact reached.

How Do CoSA Impact on the Volunteers?

Whilst efficacy research has mostly focused on the Core Members involved in CoSA, such projects would not exist or survive without members of the community volunteering their time to work with them (Bates et al., 2007; Wilson et al., 2010). It has been argued that gaining a deeper understanding of how volunteers engage the Core Members so effectively is essential (Bates et al., 2014).

The use of volunteers has also been described as the strength of CoSA, allowing Core Members to feel part of the community by having contact with 'real people' other than just professionals (Armstrong & Wills, 2014a). Indeed, the importance of using volunteers has been highlighted many times by Core Members, who believe the success of CoSA is down to involving members of the community who want to spend time with them and support them and are not being paid to do so (Hanvey et al., 2011). Despite this, until recently, very little research has focused upon the direct impact participating in CoSA has on the volunteers.

Höing, Bogaerts and Vogelvang (2015) have considered this area in detail however, focusing on a sample of 40 active volunteers on Dutch CoSA. Using a quantitative research design, volunteers were asked to complete a web based questionnaire, which explored the positive and negative aspects of being involved with CoSA. Several measures were used to examine outcomes in volunteers' satisfaction, mental wellbeing, social capital, job demands, self-esteem, external job resources and volunteer connectedness. Similar to Wilson et al. (2007a) the findings demonstrated that volunteers' main motivation for participating in CoSA was community improvement, through the reintegration of the Core Member and prevention of further sexual reoffending. This provides evidence in support of CoSA as a restorative justice initiative, a concept which is debated within the literature (see McAlinden, 2011 for more detail).

Restorative justice initiatives aim to engage offenders, in order to help them appreciate the consequences of their actions, seek reconciliation between the victim and offender, where possible, and reintegrate them back within the community (McAlinden, 2005). In CoSA, the victim is not involved directly, as is usually the case in other restorative initiatives. Despite this, it is argued that the volunteers, and therefore community's, involvement, means CoSA can be understood as a restorative intervention (see Chap. 2). This is through their disapproval of offending, encouragement of prosocial behaviour and ability to hold perpetrators of sexual crime to account (McCartan et al., 2014). In addition, victim reparation can be worked towards through the healing of fractured communities, achieved by holding offenders accountable for their offending and reasserting shared community norms (Ward, Fox, & Garber, 2014). Volunteer-led initiatives, such as CoSA empower the community to take responsibility for their own protection, and to participate in decisions about the reintegration of offenders (Bazemore & Erbe, 2004; McAlinden, 2005); behaviour, which Höing, Bogaerts and Vogelvang (2015) reported to be satisfying with positive effects on the volunteers' mental wellbeing.

An increase in social awareness as a result of volunteering for CoSA was also documented within the findings, with low levels of burnout or secondary traumatic stress. The finding of increased connectedness however, was reported as both a benefit and a risk to volunteers. Höing, Bogaerts and Vogelvang (2015) explained how an increase in connectedness can potentially blur the boundaries between the volunteers and Core Member involved, resulting in observations of risk being biased in favour of the Core Members. Although acknowledging that the dual role of connectedness and vigilance is a complex issue, they believe that this issue can be overcome through expert supervision of the volunteers by an experienced coordinator. Supervision of this nature, they argue, can ensure observations of risk are still recognised alongside support being given. Although the authors acknowledge that further research is required, the findings highlight to CoSA providers, the benefits of volunteering on a project and the importance of the role of the coordinator with regard specifically to the supervision they offer.

CoSA through the Eyes of the Public

Despite the seemingly positive benefits of CoSA for both Core Members and volunteers, it has been argued within the literature that, rather than whether society can resettle offenders on release from prison, it is more a question of whether it really wants to (Maguire & Raynor, 2006). This is even more relevant for those convicted of sexual offences who despite consistent support from CoSA volunteers, may still be faced with the stigmatization that is so prevalent in society today (Tewksbury, 2012). Indeed, Northcutt Bohmert, Duwe, and Hipple (2016) reported from their research focusing on the Minnesota CoSA programme in the US, that despite the support received, some Core Members were still unable to overcome the structural barriers to reintegration. Although only a small sample was used (n = 10 Core members), making generalisations to other CoSA projects difficult, the barriers to reintegration, which left them feeling stigmatised, were too great for some and resulted in a violation of their supervision.

To explore this area further Richards and McCartan (2017) have taken a different approach to the evaluation of CoSA, through the consideration of public perceptions of CoSA and their perceived effectiveness. They argue, this is an important area of research to consider, due to the fact that CoSA projects rely upon volunteers from the local community, therefore deeming at least some community support necessary. In addition, they acknowledge that public policy on community safety is swayed by public opinion, meaning that informing the government of the publics' views on CoSA may encourage more resources to be channelled towards the initiative. Richards and McCartan's sample consisted of individuals (n = 768) who had posted on four online social media sources, in response to the stories relating to the introduction of CoSA in Adelaide, Australia. As Richards and McCartan (2017) acknowledge, data collected from English language social media sources do not have the same representativeness expected from random samples and can result in exclusion of, for example, those who are illiterate in using online technologies or who are non-English speaking.

The results demonstrated that the majority of the individuals who had posted a comment online regarding the subject opposed the introduction of CoSA in the community. The two main reasons given for this opposition were first, a belief that the perpetrators of sexual crime did not deserve and therefore should not receive government funding. It was believed, that the resources should be spent on the victims of sexual offences instead. Second, there was a perception held, that those who offend sexually against children could not be rehabilitated and thus programs or initiatives that support this would be ineffective and a waste of resources. Some people stated that CoSA providers and supporters were 'idealistic', 'naïve' and 'do gooders' (Richards & McCartan, 2017, p. 8).

These negative views towards those who commit sexual offences are in line with the wider literature. For example, Brown, Deakin and Spencer (2008) conducted a large-scale study (n = 979) examining how individuals perceive those who commit sexual offences in the UK. From their findings, they reported that although there was a general acceptance that these individuals would return to the community, their risk of reoffending was significantly overestimated, resulting in feelings of fear, anger and anxiousness. Similar to the Richards and McCartan (2017) study, a high level of pessimism was expressed in relation to the ability for those who commit sexual offences to be rehabilitated, with a particular concern regarding such individuals living within close proximity to them. Similar results were found in Northern Ireland (2007), when exploring the potential for effective CoSA, with participants unwilling to recognise the role of the community in helping those who have previously been convicted of sexual offences to reintegrate successfully.

Although few and far between, in Richards and McCartan's (2017) study a small amount did resist the dominant view, expressing support for CoSA due to its potential to help prevent further sexual victimisation and therefore prevent future victims. The views overall however, heavily weighted towards the negative, with the majority opposing the establishment of CoSA in their community. These negative perceptions held towards those who commit sexual offences can have a detrimental impact on their successful reintegration back in to the community in terms of, for example stigmatisation and the denial of suitable housing or employment opportunities (Tewksbury, 2012). It can be argued therefore, the effectiveness of CoSA may be restricted whilst public perceptions remain as they are. Richards and McCartan (2017) acknowledge that due to these ingrained community attitudes, simply providing further information regarding the topic is unlikely to be effective in promoting positive change. They do suggest however, that community education may be more effective if delivered by the volunteers themselves who are involved in the CoSA projects; an area that is yet to be investigated. This is something that is further discussed in Chap. 6 of this book.

General Discussion: Do CoSA Work?

In conclusion, the literature to date demonstrates promising and encouraging evidence of the effectiveness of CoSA, with clear psychosocial benefits for the Core Members. Reductions in social isolation and loneliness, along with an improvement in psychological wellbeing have been reported with Core Members, both of which have positive effects on the likelihood of achieving a crime-free life. The volunteers also appear to benefit from their involvement in CoSA, although more research is required to confirm this.

Despite these results, the initiative cannot yet be considered evidence-based, due to a lack of high-quality, experimental evaluations that clearly illustrate a reduction in reoffending rates when compared to a control group (Elliott & Zajac, 2015). More controversially, Elliott (2014) has stated that the intense *wanting* of CoSA to be successful has resulted in an evidence base vulnerable to many valid and grave criticisms, which in turn may damage the initiative's credibility. Indeed, there is very little independent evidence demonstrating the effectiveness of CoSA.

Despite the mixed views of CoSA both within the literature, and from the public, there seems to be a general consensus that researchers and practitioners should remain optimistic, and continue to develop a research base that involves a thorough and comprehensive evaluation of CoSA projects (Elliott & Zajac, 2015). There have been arguments that efforts to achieve this should now be focused towards qualitative evaluations, due to the limitations to collecting ethically and statistically sound quantitative data from those who have offended sexually (McWhinnie, 2015). The following chapters will report on some of the most recent attempts at such qualitative evaluations of CoSA.

References

Aresti, A., Eatough, V., & Brooks-Gordon, B. (2010). Doing time after time: An interpretative phenomenological analysis of reformed ex-prisoners' experiences of self-change, identity and career opportunities. *Psychology, Crime & Law, 16*(3), 169–190. https://doi.org/10.1080/10683160802516273

Armstrong, S., & Wills, S. (2014a). *A review of the Fife circles of support and accountability project commissioned by SACRO—Final report*. Research report. Edinburgh: Sacro. Retrieved from www.sccjr.ac.uk

Armstrong, S., & Wills, D. (2014b). Circles of support and accountability (CoSA) in Scotland: Practice, progress and questions. *The Scottish Journal for Criminal Justice Studies, 20*, 2–13.

Bates, A., Macrae, R., Williams, D., & Webb, C. (2012). Ever-increasing circles: A descriptive study of Hampshire and Thames Valley circles of support and accountability 2002–09. *Journal of Sexual Aggression, 18*(3), 355–373. https://doi.org/10.1080/13552600.2010.544415

Bates, A., Saunders, R., & Wilson, C. (2007). Doing something about it: A follow-up study of sex offenders participating in Thames Valley circles of support and accountability. *British Journal of Community Justice, 5*(1), 19–42.

Bates, A., Williams, D., Wilson, C., & Wilson, R. J. (2014). Circles south east: The first 10 years 2002–2012. *International Journal of Offender Therapy and Comparative Criminology, 58*(7), 861–885. https://doi.org/10.1177/0306624X13485362

Bazemore, G., & Erbe, C. (2004). Reintegration and restorative justice: Towards a theory and practice of informal social control and support. In S. Maruna & R. Immarigeon (Eds.), *After crime and punishment: Pathways to offender reintegration* (pp. 27–56). Devon: Willan Publishing.

Brown, S., Deakin, J., & Spencer, J. (2008). What people think about the management of sex offenders in the community. *The Howard Journal of Crime and Justice, 47*(3), 259–274. https://doi.org/10.1111/j.1468-2311.2008.00519.x

Cann, J., Falshaw, L., & Friendship, C. (2004). Sexual offenders discharged from prison in England and Wales: A 21 year reconviction study. *Legal and Criminological Psychology, 9*(1), 1–10. https://doi.org/10.1348/135532504322776816

Duwe, G. (2012). Can circles of support and accountability (COSA) work in the United States? Preliminary results from a randomized experiment in Minnesota. *Sexual Abuse: A Journal of Research and Treatment, 25*(2), 143–165. https://doi.org/10.1177/1079063212453942

Elliott, I. (2014, June 6). CoSA: An inconvenient truth [blog post]. Retrieved from http://nextgenforensic.wordpress.com/2014/06/06/cosa-an-inconvenient-truth/

Elliott, I. A., & Beech, A. R. (2012). A UK cost-benefit analysis of circles of support and accountability interventions. *Sexual Abuse: A Journal of Research and Treatment, 25*(3), 211–229. https://doi.org/10.1177/1079063212443385

Elliott, I. A., & Zajac, G. (2015). The implementation of circles of support and accountability in the United States. *Aggression and Violent Behavior, 25*, 113–123. https://doi.org/10.1016/j.avb.2015.07.014

Elliott, I. A., Zajac, G., & Meyer, C. A. (2013). *Evaluability assessments of the circles of support and accountability (COSA) model: Cross site report*. Washington,

DC: National Institute of Justice, Office Justice Programs, US Department of Justice.

Farrall, S. (2002). *Rethinking what works with offenders: Probation, social context and desistance from crime*. Cullompton: Willan.

Fox, K. J. (2015a). Theorising community integration as desistance-promotion. *Criminal Justice and Behavior, 42*(*1*), 82–94. https://doi.org/10.1177/0093854814550028

Fox, K. J. (2015b). Contextualizing the policy and pragmatics of reintegrating sex offenders. *Sexual Abuse: A Journal of Research and Treatment*, 1–23. https://doi.org/10.1177/1079063215574711

Hannem, S. (2011). Experiences in reconciling risk management and restorative justice how circles of support and accountability work restoratively in the risk society. *International Journal of Offender Therapy and Comparative Criminology, 57*(3), 269–288. https://doi.org/10.1177/0306624x11432538

Hannem, S., & Petrunik, M. (2007). Circles of support and accountability: A community justice initiative for the reintegration of high risk sex offenders. *Contemporary Justice Review, 10*(2), 153–171. https://doi.org/10.1080/10282580701372046

Hanson, R. K. (1997). *The development of a brief actuarial risk scale for sexual offense recidivism*. User Report 97-04. Ottawa: Department of the Solicitor General of Canada.

Hanson, R. K., & Morton-Bourgon, K. E. (2005). The characteristics of persistent sexual offenders: A meta-analysis of recidivism studies. *Journal of Consulting and Clinical Psychology, 73*(6), 1154–1163. https://doi.org/10.1037/0022-006X.73.6.1154

Hanson, R. K., & Morton-Bourgon, K. E. (2009). The accuracy of recidivism risk assessments for sexual offenders: A meta-analysis of 118 prediction studies. *Psychological Assessment, 21*(1), 1–21. https://doi.org/10.1037/a0014421

Hanson, R. K., & Thornton, D. (2000). Improving risk assessments for sex offenders: A comparison of three actuarial scales. *Law and Human Behavior, 24*, 119–136. https://doi.org/10.1023/a:1005482921333

Hanvey, S., Philpot, T., & Wilson, C. (2011). *A community based approach to the reduction of sexual offending: Circles of support and accountability*. London: Jessica Kingsley Publishers.

Höing, M., Bogaerts, S., & Vogelvang, B. (2013). Circles of support and accountability: How and why they work for sex offenders. *Journal of Forensic Psychology Practice, 13*(4), 267–295. https://doi.org/10.1080/15228932.2013.808526

Höing, M., Bogaerts, S., & Vogelvang, B. (2015). Volunteers in circles of support and accountability: Job demands, job resources and outcome. *Sexual Abuse: A Journal of Research and Treatment*, 1–22. https://doi.org/10.1177/1079063215612441

Höing, M., Vogelvang, B., & Bogaerts, S. (2015). "I am a different man now"-sex offenders in circles of support and accountability: A prospective study. *International Journal of Offender Therapy and Comparative Criminology*, 1–22. https://doi.org/10.1177/0306624x15612431

LeBel, T. P., Burnett, R., Maruna, S., & Bushway, S. (2008). The chicken and egg' of subjective and social factors in desistance from crime. *European Journal of Criminology, 5*(2), 131–159. https://doi.org/10.1177/1477370807087640

Lussier, P., & Gress, C. L. (2014). Community re-entry and the path toward desistance: A quasi-experimental longitudinal study of dynamic factors and community risk management of adult sex offenders. *Journal of Criminal Justice, 42*(2), 111–122. https://doi.org/10.1016/j.jcrimjus.2013.09.006

Maguire, M., & Raynor, P. (2006). How the resettlement of prisoners promotes desistance from crime or does it? *Criminology and Criminal Justice, 6*(1), 19–38. https://doi.org/10.1177/1748895806060665

Marques, J. K., Wiederanders, M., Day, D. M., Nelson, C., & Van Ommeren, A. (2005). Effects of a relapse prevention program on sexual recidivism: Final results from California's sex offender treatment and evaluation project (SOTEP). *Sexual Abuse: A Journal of Research and Treatment, 17*(1), 79–107. https://doi.org/10.1177/107906320501700108

Marshall, W. L. (2010). The role of attachments, intimacy, and loneliness in the etiology and maintenance of sexual offending. *Sexual and Relationship Therapy, 25*(1), 73–85. https://doi.org/10.1080/14681990903550191

Marshall, W. L., & Marshall, L. E. (2007). The utility of the random controlled trial for evaluating sexual offender treatment: The gold standard or an inappropriate strategy? *Sexual Abuse: A Journal of Research and Treatment, 19*(2), 175–191. https://doi.org/10.1177/107906320701900207

McAlinden, A. (2005). The use of 'shame' with sexual offenders. *British Journal of Criminology, 45*(3), 373–394. https://doi.org/10.1093/bjc/azh095

McAlinden, A. (2011). 'Transforming justice': Challenges for restorative justice in an era of punishment-based corrections. *Contemporary Justice Review, 14*(4), 383–406. https://doi.org/10.1080/10282580.2011.616369

McCartan, K., Kemshall, H., Westwood, S., Solle, J., MacKenzie, G., & Pollard, A. (2014). Circles of Support and Accountability (CoSA): A case file review of two pilots. *Ministry of Justice Analytical Summary*. London: Ministry of Justice.

McNeill, F. (2009). What works and what's just? *European Journal of Probation, 1*(1), 21–40.

McWhinnie, A. (2015). *Circles of support in Canada*. Paper presented at the Association of the Treatment of Sexual Abusers 34th Annual Research and Treatment Conference. Montreal, QC, Canada.

Mingus, W., & Burchfield, K. B. (2012). From prison to integration: Applying modified labelling theory to sex offenders. *Criminal Justice Studies, 25*(1), 97–109. https://doi.org/10.1080/1478601X.2012.657906

Northcutt Bohmert, M. N., Duwe, G., & Hipple, N. K. (2016). Evaluating restorative justice circles of support and accountability can social support overcome structural barriers? *International Journal of Offender Therapy and Comparative Criminology*, 1–20. https://doi.org/10.1177/0306624X16652627

Paternoster, R., & Bushway, S. (2009). Desistance and the "feared self": Toward an identity theory of criminal desistance. *The Journal of Criminal Law and Criminology, 99*(4), 1103–1156.

Richards, K., & McCartan, K. (2017). Public views about reintegrating child sex offenders via circles of support and accountability (COSA): A qualitative analysis. *Deviant Behavior, 12*(5), 1–17.

Tewksbury, R. (2012). Stigmatization of sex offenders. *Deviant Behavior, 33*(8), 606–623. https://doi.org/10.1080/01639625.2011.636690

Thomas, T., Thompson, D., & K. Karstedt. (2014). *Assessing the impact of circles of support and accountability on the reintegration of adults convicted of sexual offences in the community*. Centre for Criminal Justice Studies, University of Leeds.

Thornton, D., Mann, R., Webster, S., Blud, L., Travers, R., Friendship, C., et al. (2003). Distinguishing and combining risks for sexual and violent recidivism. *Annals of the New York Academy of Sciences, 989*(1), 225–235. https://doi.org/10.1111/j.1749-6632.2003.tb07308.x

Ward, T., Fox, K. J., & Garber, M. (2014). Restorative justice, offender rehabilitation and desistance. *Restorative Justice, 2*(1), 24–42. https://doi.org/10.5235/20504721.2.1.24

Weaver, B., & McNeill, F. (2015). Lifelines desistance, social relations, and reciprocity. *Criminal Justice and Behavior, 42*(1), 95–107. https://doi.org/10.1177/0093854814550031

Wilson, C., Bates, A., & Völlm, B. (2010). Circles of support and accountability: An innovative approach to manage high-risk sex offenders in the community. *Open Criminology Journal, 3*, 48–57. https://doi.org/10.2174/1874917801003010048

Wilson, R. J., Cortoni, F., & McWhinnie, A. J. (2009). Circles of support & accountability: A Canadian national replication of outcome findings. *Sexual Abuse: A Journal of Research and Treatment, 21*(4), 412–430. https://doi.org/10.1177/1079063209347724

Wilson, R. J., & McWhinnie, A. J. (2013). Putting the "community" back in community risk management of persons who have sexually abused. *International Journal of Behavioral Consultation and Therapy, 8*(3-4), 72–79. https://doi.org/10.1037/h0100987

Wilson, R. J., McWhinnie, A. J., & Wilson, C. (2008). Circles of support and accountability: An international partnership in reducing sexual offender recidivism. *Prison Service Journal, 138*, 26–36.

Wilson, R. J., Picheca, J. E., & Prinzo, M. (2005). *Circles of support and accountability: An evaluation of the pilot project in South-Central Ontario*. Ottawa, ON: Correctional Service of Canada.

Wilson, R. J., Picheca, J. E., & Prinzo, M. (2007a). Evaluating the effectiveness of professionally facilitated volunteerism in the community based management of high risk sexual offenders: Part One–Effects on participants and stakeholders. *The Howard Journal of Criminal Justice, 46*(3), 289–302. https://doi.org/10.1111/j.1468-2311.2007.00475.x

Wilson, R. J., Picheca, J. E., & Prinzo, M. (2007b). Evaluating the effectiveness of professionally facilitated volunteerism in the community based management of high risk sexual offenders: Part Two–A comparison of the recidivism rates. *The Howard Journal of Criminal Justice, 46*(4), 327–337. https://doi.org/10.1111/j.1468-2311.2007.00480.x

4

The Prison-Based Model of Circles of Support and Accountability and its Application in Transitioning to the Community

Rosie Kitson-Boyce

Introduction

In society today, those who commit sexual crimes are portrayed negatively and sensationally by the media, often provoking anger, fear and even hatred towards them from the general public (McAlinden, 2006). It is widely established within the literature that individuals who have been convicted of sexual offences face increased levels of stress, difficulties in finding employment and housing, and problems maintaining social and familial relationships (Tewksbury, 2012; Tewksbury & Connor, 2012; Tewksbury & Copes, 2013). These barriers to successful reintegration often lead to social isolation and prevent desistance from crime being achieved (Tewksbury & Mustaine, 2009).

Göbbels, Ward, and Willis (2012) expand on this further stating that, negative social capital, such as the loss of relationships, inability to gain employment or housing and stigmatisation (Lussier & Gress, 2014;

R. Kitson-Boyce (✉)
Nottingham Trent University, Nottingham, UK

H. Elliott et al. (eds.), *Sexual Crime and Circles of Support and Accountability*, Sexual Crime, https://doi.org/10.1007/978-3-319-74823-8_4

Tewksbury, 2012), can be barriers to successful re-entry in to the community for those convicted of sexual offences. They point out that even ex-offenders who have worked hard to undergo significant identity changes do not always re-enter communities that reinforce these new non-offender identities. In addition, the lack of support those who commit sexual offences receive during this transitional period from prison to community makes the process difficult and uncertain (Elliott & Zajac, 2015).

This is concerning due to the early stages of release being a particularly sensitive period in terms of achieving this desistance (Aresti, Eatough, & Brooks-Gordon, 2010). Furthermore, when considering the wellbeing of offenders recently released from prison, Fox (2015) acknowledged how individuals can quickly become overwhelmed, particularly if they have served a long sentence in prison. Interestingly, Van den Berg, Beijersbergen, Nieuwbeerta, and Dirkzwager (2017) reported from their sample of Dutch offenders that there was no difference between those who were convicted of sexual offences and those convicted of all other offences, in terms of their level of loneliness whilst in prison. Upon release therefore, the differential negative treatment those convicted of sexual offences receive once in the community, could lead to even further feelings of overwhelm and maybe even shock.

One suggestion Göbbels et al. (2012) make to assist those convicted of sexual offences through the transition of re-entry is artificial mentoring. An artificial mentor they argue, is someone who can provide social modelling to the individual but also sustained and empathetic support to promote and encourage the motivation to maintain desistance. The volunteers who are involved in CoSA may be able to take on this role of a mentor. They can offer support to the Core Member, helping them maintain their non-offender identity but also encouraging them to build social networks outside of the CoSA, which verify the ex-offender's change in identity and behaviour. The CoSA model however, is a community one, meaning that support for the Core Member commences once they have been released into the community, sometimes with delays of several weeks (Höing, Vogelvang, & Bogaerts, 2015). This therefore requires the Core Members, who are normally experiencing a severe lack of social support, to still transition from prison to the community alone.

A prison-based model of CoSA however, can provide 'Through the Gate' support to those convicted of sexual offences as will now be considered in more detail.

Early Prison-Based CoSA

A project that has successfully implemented a continuum of support from prison to the community for individuals convicted of sexual offences, is MnCoSA in the US. In 2008, MnCoSA was implemented in Minnesota, US, involving individuals convicted of sexual offences who were due to be released from prison. As Duwe (2012) explains, MnCoSA developed from the promising results of Wilson, Picheca, and Prinzo's (2005) initial evaluation study, with the design and operation being very similar to that of the Canadian CoSA. One fundamental difference however, was that unlike in Canada whereby CoSA begins after the offender has been released from prison, MnCoSA was systematically designed to begin at least four weeks prior to the offender's release (Duwe, 2012). Offered through the Minnesota Department of Corrections, MnCoSA focuses upon the successful transition from prison to community for individuals convicted for sexual offences (MnCoSA, 2017). The volunteers meet with the Core Member approximately three times whilst in prison before the sessions move in to the community as the Core Member re-enters society (MnCoSA, 2017).

Duwe (2012) highlights the importance of the continuum of social support from prison to community and believes it to be a central factor in why MnCoSA has been successful in reintegrating those who commit sexual offences back in to the community (see the previous chapter for more detail on his RCT of MnCoSA). Indeed, Maguire and Raynor (2006) believe that for offenders to re-settle effectively on release, through care is needed involving the establishment of a close relationship with the offender while they are still in prison, which is then continued in release. It is believed that this relationship should be well-established, involve trust and a willingness to travel together on the path towards desistance (McNeill & Weaver, 2010).

When considering offenders, who are still residing in prison, Rocque, Biere, and MacKenzie (2011) have highlighted how increasing the attachment and improving social bonds to prosocial individuals results in a positive outcome. Within their study, attachment and social bonds were defined as a feeling of closeness to significant others, with their impact on the intention to conform being explored. For individuals who have committed sexual offences, achieving and developing an attachment or social bond with members of the community is difficult, particularly when family and friends may have cut ties due to the nature of their crime or restraining orders are in place preventing contact (Lussier & Gress, 2014). This therefore highlights a need for the prison-based model of CoSA.

It is important to consider however, that the volunteers involved in a prison-based model of CoSA will have met the old (criminal) self as well as the new desisting self. It is argued that to desist from crime successfully, offenders need to develop a new pro-social identity separate to their past self (Maruna, 2001). It is therefore possible that some potential Core Members will want to leave their past behind completely and not want to be involved with anyone who knew them during their past life. As Serin and Lloyd (2009) point out however, desistance from crime takes time, with the offender gradually committing themselves to prosocial lifestyles. They go on to explain that because of this there will be a transitional period whereby the offender and the ex-offender overlap. The MnCoSA, unlike the community model of CoSA, can provide social support to the Core Member through this transitional stage, thus in turn encouraging and motivating them to continue on their journey to desistance.

CoSA: The UK Prison-Based Model

In 2014, the first ever UK prison-based model of CoSA was established at HMP Whatton, a category-C treatment prison for individuals convicted of a sexual offence who are prepared to address their offending behaviour through participation in a treatment programme. This was the first time CoSA that began in the prison, before moving out in to the community, had been operationalised in the UK.

The CoSA prison-based model initiative was set up by the Safer Living Foundation (SLF); a charitable organisation involving employees from the prison, Nottingham Trent University, probation and police. There was a concern felt by the trustees of the SLF that some individuals serving sentences for sexual offences, particularly those who were elderly (55+) or who had intellectual disabilities (ID), were leaving prison without any family or community support. Individuals with ID who commit sexual offences have received a specific focus within the literature, with ID often being described as overrepresented amongst this group of offenders (Hayes, Shackell, Mottram, & Lancaster, 2007; Lambrick & Glaser, 2004). Indeed, Craig and Hutchinson (2005) calculated that the reconviction rate for ID offenders convicted of a sexual offence was 6.8 times at two years follow up, and 3.5 times at four years to that of non-ID offenders convicted of similar sexual offences. It must be acknowledged however, that the research on this group of individuals is extremely flawed, with methodological differences between the studies being so great that conclusions regarding the true prevalence of sexual offences by men with ID are difficult to state (Craig & Hutchinson, 2005; Lindsay, 2002). With regard to elderly individuals who commit sexual offences, the decrease in societal tolerance, along with a greater readiness for the police and prosecutors to pursue and secure more 'late-in-life' convictions for non-recent sexual offences has seen a growth in the amount of elderly individuals in prison for a sexual offence (Crawley & Sparks, 2005; Hart, 2008). For example, in 2006, Fazel, Sjöstedt, Långström and Grann reported that around half of all male offenders aged 60+ in England and Wales were serving custodial sentences for a sexual offence.

In addition to both groups being highly represented within prison settings, elderly and ID men are particularly vulnerable during the transition from prison to community (Crawley & Sparks, 2006; Cummins & Lau, 2003). For elderly offenders, the fear of isolation on release can be even greater, with many nursing homes and elderly care facilities reluctant to accept these individuals due to the type of offences they have committed (Hart, 2008). Individuals with ID are reported to have a lack of social networks and resultant lack of feelings of connectedness, both of which are required for successful community integration (Cummins & Lau, 2003). This, combined with a severe lack of social support on release, means social isolation is almost inevitable for elderly and ID offenders. Loneliness and isolation, often caused by problematic or unsuccessful reintegration, can exacerbate the risk of reoffending for those convicted of sexual offences (Clarke, Brown, & Völlm, 2015; Fox, 2015). It was acknowledged therefore, that a continuum of support was needed for these individuals, through the transition from prison to community, thus leading to the establishment of the first UK prison-based model of CoSA.

This prison-based CoSA focuses on individuals convicted of a sexual offence with determinate prison sentences (i.e. a fixed release date) who were elderly (55+) or intellectually disabled (ID) and were deemed medium to very high static risk using the RM2000 risk assessment tool (Thornton et al., 2003). There is no universal definition of 'elderly', however within criminal justice literature, 'older' is defined as starting anywhere between 45 and 65 years (Bows & Westmarland, 2016). Most US research on offenders use 50 as the starting point for the 'older' category, which Howse (2003) suggests may be the point at which offenders begin to view themselves as 'old'. In the UK, 50 is also used in some cases as the age at which someone is classed as older, for example Evergreen 50+, a project to support older prisoners in England and Wales. Until recently, retirement age in the UK was 65 (Gov.uk, 2017). However, as Howse (2003) acknowledged in his report for the Prison Reform Trust, individuals residing in a prison setting tend to have a biological age of 10 years older than individuals in the community, due to their chronic health problems. Bows and Westmarland (2016) have more recently agreed, stating that the mental and physical health problems offenders in prison experience results in a more rapid onset of age related issues, compared to their counterparts outside prison. This provides an argument for a lower threshold for an 'elderly' category and indeed Age UK, the largest charity in the UK to work with older individuals including prisoners, have 55 as the starting age of their 'elderly' category. Based on these considerations, the prison-based model of CoSA determined 55 to be a suitable age at which individuals could be considered for a Core Member place. Individuals were also required to have little to no social support on release, due to the increased risk these individuals pose on release.

The CoSA in the UK prison-based model begin around three months prior to the Core Member's release from prison and continue with the Core Member for up to 12 months in the community. The volunteers visit the prison weekly for the CoSA meetings whilst the Core Member is still residing there and are therefore required to undergo criminal security checks before beginning their role. The CoSA meetings continue through the transitional period from prison to community, with the meetings continuing in the first week of the Core Member's release. Once in the community the CoSA meetings can take place at either the approved premises the Core Member is being housed at, the SLF offices at Nottingham Trent University, or in certain situations nearby Quaker rooms or the Core Members' own home.

Prison Model Evaluation

As has been outlined above, a prison-based model of CoSA provides potential positive benefits for those convicted of sexual offences in the UK. In particular, those who are categorised as elderly or ID and are facing release from prison with a severe lack of social support. It is crucial that any new process, such as the prison-based model being established in the UK, is evaluated from its commencement. As the previous chapter outlined, there have been substantial criticisms of the quantitative data reported from CoSA research. Clarke et al. (2015) have stated that, whilst good quality evaluations of recidivism are important, they do not capture the full extent of the impact participating in CoSA can have. This has led to a demand for qualitative studies involving the Core Members and volunteers taking part in CoSA (Bates, Williams, Wilson, & Wilson, 2014; Wilson, Bates, & Völlm, 2010).

A qualitative evaluation was therefore commenced at the same time the UK prison-based model of CoSA began, involving interviews with the Core Members to explore their personal experience of the prison-based model. The rest of this chapter will explore some of the key themes derived from the data in relation to the support the prison-based model of CoSA provided the Core Members during their transition from prison to community.

Demographics

The Core Member places on the prison-based model of CoSA were allocated according to a number of criteria. These are briefly outlined below, along with the main demographic details of the participants within this research.

Conviction for sexual offence. The first criterion was that the individual must have committed a sexual offence and currently be residing in the prison where the CoSA prison-based model was established. Offence histories of the participants were predominantly of contact sexual offences against children. The skew towards this offence history is relative to the general population at the prison the participants were recruited from.

Elderly or intellectually disabled. The second criterion was that these individuals must ideally either be elderly or be defined as having an intellectual disability. Using the IQ tests already carried out by the prison in order to determine treatment suitability, individuals were considered as a potential Core Member if they had an IQ of >80 or were over the age of 55 years. Using an IQ of below 80 ensured those with borderline ID were also considered for a place. However, for individuals whose IQ was in the borderline range, an Adaptive Functioning Checklist (AFC) (created by Dr Lorraine Smith at Nottingham Trent University) was also used to assess adaptive and social functioning. Forty percent of the participants included in the research were defined as having mild-borderline ID and 80% were 55 years of age or older (see Table 4.1).

Risk of reoffending. It was essential that the resources of the CoSA prison-based model were allocated to those who were most at risk of recidivism. The most widely used actuarial risk assessment tool in the English and Wales prison and probation services is the Risk Matrix 2000 (RM2000; Thornton et al., 2003). This risk assessment tool measures static risk of reoffending and is used to help inform decisions about appropriate treatment pathways and management of offenders in the community. As Barnett, Wakeling, and Howard (2010) state, the use of such assessment tools enables effective allocation of resources to

Table 4.1 Core Member participant information

Participant number	Participant age	Intellectual disability	Health issues	Risk level (RM2000)
1	60	Yes—mild	Yes—physical	Medium
2	60	No	Yes—physical	Medium
3	60	Yes—mild	Yes—physical	Very high
4	45	Borderline	No	Medium
5	58	No	Yes—mental	Medium
6	78	No	Yes—physical and mental	Medium
7	73	No	No	Very high
8	64	Yes—mild	No	High
9	52	No	No	Very high

those at a higher risk of reoffending and the same applies for the prison-based model of CoSA. Using the RM2000, 60 percent of the participants involved in the research were assessed as a medium risk of sexual reoffending, 10 percent were placed in the high risk category and 30 percent in the very high risk category (see Table 4.1).

Individuals who had been offered and accepted a Core Member place on a prison-based model CoSA (December 2014–August 2016) were approached regarding their participation in the research project. Those who consented were asked to participate in data collection at three time points during their CoSA prison-based model journey, as shown in Table 4.2.

As stated previously the prison-based model of CoSA in the UK is designed to begin approximately three months before the Core Members release from prison. This process is flexible however and varies with each individual CoSA, as can be seen in Table 4.3 below. There are several reasons for this, with the main one being that a referral for a potential Core Member with high need may not be received by the coordinator until later in their sentence. As is stated above however, in the US prison-model of CoSA, the volunteers meet with the Core Member only three times before their release. This still provides enough time for a social bond to at least have begun to be developed, thus providing additional support over the transitional period of release as is highlighted in the findings below.

Table 4.2 Time point of data collection with Core Members

Time point	Position in the CoSA prison-based model journey	*N*
1	Prior to the Core Member meeting the volunteers involved in their CoSA	9
2	After the prison sessions of the CoSA, just before release into the community	6
3	Once in the community but still taking part in the CoSA	7

Table 4.3 Planned and actual number of prison CoSA sessions

Participant number	Planned time for prison sessions	Actual number of prison sessions
1	2 months, 1 week	6
2	2 weeks	2
3	3 months, 2 weeks	7
4	1 month, 1 week	6
5	1 month	4
6	1 month	3
7	IPP sentence (parole date not confirmed)	IPP sentence (parole date not confirmed)
8	3 weeks	2
9	1 month, 2 weeks	6

Transition from Prison to Community

The purpose of this research was to explore the experiences of the Core Members throughout their journey on a prison-based model of CoSA. As stated previously, data was collected at three different time points to capture their transition from prison to community.

Data Collection

Semi-structured interviews were chosen as the method for data collection, to capture both the richness and complexity of the individuals' experience (Aresti et al., 2010). Semi-structured interviews involve a set of questions used by the researcher to guide the interview, rather than dictate it, meaning the participant is viewed as the expert on the topic discussed (Smith & Osborn, 2003). In addition, due to the participants potentially having ID, the interview schedules were written in suitable language with a Felsch readability score of 2.9. This meant the questions posed could be understood by an individual with the reading ability of a seven year old and therefore suitable to be used with those who had borderline to mild ID.

Each interview lasted on average 1–1.5 hours. Questions for the Core Members explored their expectations and aspirations for the future. Example questions included: 'What do you think it will be like when you leave prison?', 'Who will be there to support/help you when you leave prison?', 'What were the good/bad things about being in a circle when you moved from prison to the community?'.

Analysis

The interviews were analysed using Interpretative Phenomenological Analysis (IPA) which is concerned with a detailed examination of the individuals' subjective experience (Brocki & Wearden, 2006); in this case their experience of being involved in a prison-based model CoSA. Several themes were derived from the data regarding the support a prison-based model of CoSA could provide to the Core Members during their transition from prison to the community, as are highlighted in Table 4.4.

The following analysis will explore and unpack these themes in detail to provide a rich understanding of the participants' experiences on a

Table 4.4 Themes from the interview data with corresponding data collection time points

Theme	Time point (T)
Knowing they will have support	1
Building relationships	1, 2
Preparation	2
Immediate support	3
Barriers to successful reintegration	3

prison-based model of CoSA. For further discussion of the findings from the research project discussed here, see Kitson-Boyce, Blagden, Winder, and Dillon (2018a, 2018b).

Findings

Knowing They Will Have Support

The first theme was derived from the data collected prior to the CoSA starting in the prison (T1). The Core Members identified that, aside from the prison-based CoSA, they would have little to no support on release from prison.

> They (prison-based model coordinator) approached me yeah because I haven't got any erm support network out there at all, there's no family, friends or anything. (CM Participant 2, T1)

Here the Core Member is explaining how he is facing a life in the community with no friends or family to support him, a situation that is not uncommon for those convicted of sexual offences (Tewksbury & Copes, 2013). This is particularly concerning due to the research demonstrating loneliness and social isolation as risk factors of sexual reoffending (Hanson & Morton-Bourgon, 2005; Marshall, 2010). The Core Members involved in the prison-based model recognised that individuals with a severe lack of pro-social support on release from prison are prioritised for CoSA and were aware of the potential benefits being involved could offer.

> I realised that circles offers you something that some people get from their families but if you've no family err or not in contact with your family, you've not support out there. (CM participant 9, T1)

Here the Core Member explains how for him, a prison-based model CoSA would go some way to providing the support that others may receive from their families, both whilst in prison and once released back into the community. This is particularly important due to the role social support provided by family members can provide in reducing the likelihood of future criminal behaviour on release from prison (Willis & Grace, 2008). For example, from their research into social ties, re-entry and recidivism, Berg and Huebner (2011) found that good quality ties to relatives, and the social support they provided was what motivated ex-offenders to reintegrate back into society successfully and live a pro-social life. As the Core Member acknowledged however, such support does not always have to be provided through family relations. Weaver and McNeill (2015) reported from their research that the social relations influential in supporting desistance could be friendship groups and faith communities, as well as families. It was the sense of solidarity and 'we-ness' that characterised these social relations that assisted the ex-offender in realising their pro social aspirations the most. With this in mind, it is possible that the social support offered through a prison-based model CoSA may be enough to encourage and promote desistance from Core Members.

As explained in the previous chapter (and Chap. 2), CoSA can provide benefits to communities through the reduction of potential future victims. In addition to this however, the findings demonstrate how the prison-based model CoSA can provide benefits to the Core Members also. Knowing they would have the support of the CoSA leads to improvement in their wellbeing, particularly due to the knowledge that this support will come from 'normal' members of the community.

> The support, knowing there was that amount of support out there for me, you know, just a like sad, lonely old git you know with nowhere to go, suddenly I don't need to bury my head in the sand, I know there's people there to support me, so from that point of view I feel a lot more confident. (CM Participant 5, T1)

> Because you know, they're volunteers, they come all this way to see a prisoner but they want to come and see you for a purpose…we talked a lot about it and it's wonderful. (CM Participant 7, T1)

As the last extract in particular highlights, having someone to talk to who is not a professional appears important to the Core Members. The volunteers are not paid to work with Core Members; they are there because they choose to be, resulting in their actions being perceived as genuine. Indeed, research in to the perceptions of those who commit sexual offences have concluded that the publics' attitude is generally negative and punitive towards this group of offenders (Levenson, Brannon, Fortney, & Baker, 2007). It is unsurprising therefore that having 'normal' members of the community meet with them on a weekly basis with a non-judgemental attitude is viewed so positively for Core Members.

This theme is consistent with research on CoSA in general, whereby Core Members attribute the success of CoSA to the involvement of members of the community who are 'not doing it to get paid, it's something they wanna do' (Hanvey, Philpot, & Wilson, 2011, p. 105). Similarly, Thomas, Thompson, and Karstedt (2014, p. 194) reported, from their interviews with Core Members on a community CoSA, that having 'normal people' who were able to see past their offences was 'life-changing' for the individuals. This is an important finding; if the volunteers' actions and behaviours are perceived as genuine then they are more likely to be successful in reinforcing any emerging pro-social narratives that are essential for desistance to be achieved (King, 2013).

This acknowledgement and acceptance from the Core Members of the support the CoSA will offer them, along with the perceived genuineness of the volunteers' actions, enables rapport and subsequent relationships to be built, as will now be discussed.

Building Relationships

Even from the data derived from time point 1, it was evident that the prison sessions would be beneficial in providing time and space for relationships to be built between Core Members and volunteers, before the reality of re-entering the community set in. Prior to starting the prison-based model CoSA, all but one of the Core Members interviewed stated that they were nervous and wary of meeting the volunteers.

> Cause it feels like, how do I explain it, you're in a room like this and you feel a bit nervous cause I don't know them and they don't know them and I'll be a bit on edge, a bit thinking 'are you judging me or something. (CM Participant 4, T1)

The Core Member here describes being wary, nervous and on edge until he has had the time and opportunity to get to know his volunteers. Due to the Core Members currently being in prison, the highly sensational media representation of those who commit sexual offences and the anger and hatred felt towards them (McAlinden, 2006) is likely to be their view of the general public as a whole. As Nellis (2009) explains, the stereotype the media has created, of those who commit sexual offences completely overlooks those who are motivated to start new lives and desist from sexually reoffending. This leads to the question therefore of whether Core Members, particularly those who have high levels of paranoia or low levels of self-esteem, are more likely to make the step to meet the volunteers whilst they are still in the safety of a prison setting. Although more research is required to compare directly the prison-model with the community model, in the prison-based model at least, the Core Members viewed meeting the volunteers whilst they were still in their 'comfort zone' as a positive aspect to their experience. This meant rapport and relationships could be built, and any nervousness overcome, whilst they still felt in a 'safe' environment.

> Well I'm in comfortable surroundings, I've got used to this place, it's my comfort zone so it will be ideal for me, you know I can always retreat back in (to my cell), sort of thing so I've got my comfort zone, out there it could be a bit more difficult, a bit more erm cause it's going to be a whole shock to the system, I've been in prison now nearly 6 years, there's a lot changed out there, it's going to be quite a shock to the system going out on my own and no support apart from my probation officer. (CM Participant 2, T1)

Here, the Core Member is explaining how it would be more difficult to meet a group of volunteers and begin to form relationships with them on release from prison, particularly considering the institutionalisation he is likely to have experienced from being in prison for several years. Despite this demonstrating the benefit of the prison model, the nature of the establishment where this CoSA project is taking place cannot be overlooked. A prison sentence for someone convicted of a sexual offence is often characterised by stigmatisation, feelings of anxiety and fear of being 'ousted' as a 'sexual offender' (Schwaebe, 2005). Even when segregated on a vulnerable offenders' wing, those convicted of sexual offences have reported physically frightening events, such as having insults and objects thrown at them, resulting in damaged self-esteem (Ievins, 2013). The prison in focus here however, is one of the largest sex offender treatment prisons in Europe, specialising in both rehabilitative programmes and sex offender treatment, and only housing those convicted of sexual offences. The prison has been described by offenders themselves as a place of acceptance, generating a feeling of safety they had never experienced before (Blagden, Winder, & Hames, 2016; Ievins, 2013). This feeling of being 'safe' and the reduction in anxiety has been documented as creating additional 'head space' for the offenders to reflect upon the self, work through problems and contemplate change. This leads to the question therefore of whether similar prison-based models of CoSA would work as beneficially under different circumstances. For example, in a prison whereby potential Core Members were held on a separate vulnerable prisoner's wing. Or indeed, whether the need for this type of project would be even greater.

By the time the Core Members were about to transition from prison and re-enter the community (T2) the dynamics of the CoSA had begun to settle.

> I: How do you feel about the meetings as they've been going on then, leading up to each meeting, how does it make you feel?
>
> P: it's making me feel, how can I explain it, a bit more relaxed and slowly I'm starting to build up that relationship and also that trust and that's how it's gotta be. (CM Participant 4, T2)

Here you can see how the prison sessions enabled relationships and trust to be built between the Core Member and their volunteers, overcoming the nervousness and anxiety they previously expressed during timepoint 1. By the time the CoSA moves into the community the Core Members feel more comfortable with the volunteers, enabling deeper discussions to take place. Research that has considered how probation officers are best able to assist ex-offenders in the desistance process highlights the importance of relationships involving this type of rapport (Barry, 2007). Ex-offenders are reported as being more receptive to direct guidance from probation officers when relationships are formed through receptively listening to one another (McCulloch, 2005). This highlights the benefit of the Core Members having established relationships with the volunteers prior to release, as they are more likely to accept the support and guidance towards desistance once in the community.

In addition to building rapport, all those involved in the prison-based model CoSA had the opportunity to learn and practice how to work effectively with one another so that they could 'hit the ground running' in the community. This links specifically with the next theme of preparation; providing the Core Members with additional time to build relationships with the volunteers also enabled preparation for life on release to begin.

Preparation

The data derived from the second time point highlighted how, in relation to offence related behaviour specifically, the prison sessions were used by the volunteers to help prepare the Core Members for possible risky situations on release, and to discuss management strategies in relation to their restrictions. For some Core Members, this involved acting out role-plays for the potential risky situations, for example if they came across an injured child in the street and there was no one else around.

> It's like if a little gal got knocked over by a car obviously I would phone the police and let them deal with it, cause I wouldn't go up and touch her cause if I did that and then the police knew I'd just come out of prison for a sex offence well I'd be back in again wouldn't I so I'd phone the police or if there was somebody else walking by I'd tell them to get the police, I mean I'd stop well away. It's like one instance you know I take the dog on the park, what happens if the kids come up and stroke the dog and I said 'well you know, all I've got to say to the kids, is do not stroke the dog cause I don't want the dog to bite you' and I'll just carry on walking, you know and stuff like that and err I got it all right, it was stuff like that so you know that's one thing I've got out of it (the prison sessions of the CoSA). (CM Participant 1, T2)

Here the participant is highlighting how the prison sessions are helping to prepare for situations he may face on release. Integrated within his concerns for release is an anxiety regarding the stigmatisation he will face for being convicted of a sexual offence; the police would believe his actions to have a sexual motive. This issue of stigmatisation on release is explored in more detail in the final theme of this chapter.

> so like I knew my what I've got to and what I aint got to do but when I went back, I was thinking all the time and I said to them, I says well 'where I live', I says 'it's about half an hours walk up to the town' but up at the top of the town you've got outside toilets, ladies and gents and there's many a time I've passed there when I've gone shopping with my partner, daughter, many a times I've gone up town, had a cup of tea in a café and have a walk round the market and that and I've come out and I've told them that I've got a weak bladder, I've only got to drink what a cup of water and I'm running to the toilet and I went to these toilets, ladies and gents obviously I went in to the gents but I could hear kids, I could see little lads like that (shows how tall they were) and I've seen them day in, day out, day in, day out and they have these balloons, you can buy these balloons and you fill they up with water and they chuck them at each other and I turned round and I said 'well say for instance you know I've done me shopping and that and I said to me wife, wait there and I'm just going to the toilet', I said 'can I go to that toilet where the little lads are or do I have to wait outside and pee myself or if I want to have a sit down. (Core Member Participant 1, T2)

This extract illuminates how discussing the Core Members' licence conditions during the prison sessions ensured that they understood areas or situations they would be restricted from on release. This was a particular benefit to those Core Members assessed as having ID, due to their tendency to feign understanding. For example, individuals with ID may acquiesce when not understanding questions asked, due to both their cognitive impairment and also their desire to comply socially with the perceived demands of an authority figure (Shaw & Budd, 1982). In the case of the extract above, the participant (who was assessed as ID) had read that he could not use public toilets when they were occupied by children on release but did not fully understand the details of this.

The prison sessions enabled in depth discussions to ensure this was understood clearly including what he could do instead should the situation arise.

> Err explaining things to me in a different light, how I deal with like err somethings I don't grab and they're on about doing like role-plays, I don't mind doing that, they talk to me and everything so that's a good thing. (CM Participant 4, T2)

Here the Core Member is explaining how the volunteers helped him to understand information by explaining it in a different way. Individuals with ID often experience a range of cognitive deficits, which can affect the way they process information, for example, concentration on and comprehension of what is being said to individuals with ID is likely to be limited (Craig & Hutchinson, 2005). The volunteer training for the prison-based model of CoSA involves specific guidance for how to work most effectively with these individuals. For example, breaking information down into small chunks, reducing the speed of what is being said and the use of pictures and drawings to help explain complex concepts (Craig & Hutchinson, 2005). The above extract indicates that the guidance appears to have been taken on board by the volunteers and being used effectively in the prison sessions.

Some Core Members were even able to reach the point where they were comfortable in discussing the coping strategies they use to manage offence related thoughts and feelings, often learnt previously on Sex Offender Treatment Programmes.

> I took all my stuff from HSP and they read it and so on, it was lovely to disclose it. You know it makes you feel better, you don't hide anything inside yourself and you think 'ooh what will they think of me if I tell them what I've done' and so on but none of that, they were superb. (CM Participant 7, T2)

Here the Core Member highlights the benefits of disclosing his previous offence related thoughts and behaviour. It appears that the absence of judgement from volunteers, even after sharing his darkest thoughts, and the behaviour that evolved from them, enables him to feel accepted rather than vilified as is so often the case in society today (McAlinden, 2006). Not only are the volunteers able to reinforce the Core member's use of coping strategies to successfully manage offence-related thoughts and behaviour, by offering acceptance and inclusion upon hearing this information they are in fact reinforcing this new pro-social identity also (Weaver & McNeill, 2015).

The preparation for and practicing of their new, pro social identity highlighted in this theme, encourages the Core Member to become accountable for their own thoughts and behaviour, even before they are released from prison. Both the additional support and encouraged accountability offered through the prison sessions can continue with the Core Member through the transitional period of release into the community, as is discussed in the following theme.

Immediate Support

The prison-based model of CoSA enables the Core Members involved to be supported through the transitional period of release, whereby they move from prison into the community. The Core Members discussed their appreciation for the support they received immediately on release, particularly for those re-settling in an area that is new to them.

> I mean **** (one of the volunteers) picked me up from prison so he bought me to the hostel so they had some hands on straight away. (Core Member Participant 6, T3)

> Participant: "Erm a good base, I think when you come out you need a base and if you're away, like me away from family and I think that's one of the important things, it has it's been a good consistent base to get me kind of kick started."
>
> Interviewer: "How did it make you feel having those volunteers off the train?"
>
> Participant: "It was good because we'd already met inside **** (prison) I think we met for 6 months inside before so it was good to have a couple of familiar faces… I think the bond needs to be there before you leave prison

> because if it's not there, if you're not fully committed before you leave then there's always a chance that someone might just say no it's not working on the outside. You won't be committed unless you're bonded and you need that bond on the inside I think. (CM Participant 10, T3)

In the case of these participants, the volunteers were able to meet the Core Member on their first day of release from prison and go with them to their hostel. Due to the relationships already formed in the prison sessions, as have been described earlier, the Core Member felt comforted, by 'familiar faces', in a situation that could easily have created anxiety. Interestingly Core Member 10 describes the bond he had formed with the volunteers whilst in prison and how this gave him a base to 'kick start' him in to the crime-free life he hoped to achieve. Those convicted of sexual offences routinely find it difficult to form social bonds with members of the community (Lussier & Gress, 2014). The relationships developed within the prison-based model of CoSA however, enabled a sense of support and togetherness to be present immediately on release from prison. In turn, these social bonds are argued to have a positive impact on the individual's motivation to achieve desistance (Weaver & McNeill, 2015).

> with the group yeah I found them very supportive, they were always there straight away swapping phone numbers and stuff like that and then they explained to me who was going to be on duty that weekend you know if anything happened I could get in touch with them and they're still doing that now. (Core Member Participant 2, T3)

Here the participant is highlighting how the volunteers met him immediately on release and explained how someone would be on call all weekend if he needed support; his first weekend in the community after 6 years in prison. Providing support immediately on release from prison is vital, due to an increased risk to individuals recently re-entering the community. For example, a fifth (21%) of suicides in the first year taking place during the first 28 days (Pratt, Piper, Appleby, Webb, & Shaw, 2006). As Tewksbury and Connor (2012) concluded from their research however, when positive, stable and pro-social relationships are provided to those convicted of sexual offences, both while in prison and upon re-entering society, a sense of belonging is created and law-abiding conduct promoted.

Rather than focus on the additional support for the Core Members however, CoSA have been criticised in the literature for attempting, through the use of volunteers, to provide statutory supervision 'on the cheap' (Armstrong, Chistyakova, Mackenzie, & Malloch, 2008). From this perspective a prison-based model of CoSA would provide additional supervision during the early stages of release; a particularly sensitive period in terms of risk of reoffending (Aresti et al., 2010). This is strongly contested by CoSA organisations (Thomas, Thompson, & Karstedt, 2014). Although CoSA within the UK support risk management through the accountability element, they do not duplicate or seek to replace statutory supervision of those convicted of sexual offences released from prison. Instead, they aim to complement and work in addition to the supervision that already exists for these individuals in the community (McCartan, Kemshall, Westwood, MacKenzie & Pollard, 2014). McCartan (2015) supported this, stating that all those involved in CoSA internationally must remember that volunteers are indeed volunteers and not probation officers; the aim of CoSA is not solely risk management, support also reduces the risk of reoffending.

Barriers to Successful Reintegration

As outlined previously, those who commit sexual offences face considerable barriers to successful reintegration when released from prison. For the Core Members interviewed in this research, three main issues reported were: problems finding suitable housing, health concerns and perceived stigmatisation.

With regard to the first issue, all of the Core Members interviewed reported problems securing suitable (i.e. for mobility issues) and permanent (i.e. not an approved premises) housing on release from prison.

> Oh I've been messed about with **** (housing association) from the word go. (Participant 2, T3)

> *P:* "(Probation) not letting me look for accommodation when I've already proved I can hold tenancy for two years, I think it's just not justified stopping me doing that...."
> I: "How long have you got left there?"
> P: "I don't know, obviously I'm in their hands now. I can't look for places."
> I: "Is it the same area, they're going to keep you in ****?"
> P: "I really don't know, no body's interviewed me from **** or **** or you know, the only thing he's said is I can start looking for places after about 6 months in either **** or ****. (CM Participant 8, T3)

Here the Core Members are expressing their frustrations regarding their accommodation, creating feelings of restriction and of being unsettled. In addition, Willis and Grace (2008) have argued that factors such as low quality accommodation are specifically related to reoffending. In relation to this, Northcutt Bohmert, Duwe, and Hipple (2016) documented from their study on CoSA in the US that Core Members struggled to overcome the barriers to finding housing deemed suitable by the courts, which in some cases resulted in the Core Member returning to prison.

Although CoSA are not involved directly with housing organisations, the volunteers were able to provide the Core Members with a safe space to vent their frustrations. With regard to the effectiveness of CoSA Northcutt Bohmert et al. (2016) defined this type of 'friendship' and expressive support offered by the volunteers as critical in terms of CoSA success. Expressive support is harder for the Core Members to access without the support of the CoSA and as has been evidenced previously in this chapter, the participants valued having 'normal', non-professional individuals to talk to greatly.

In addition, the CoSA sessions provided an opportunity to discuss pro-active behaviour the Core Members can engage in, in order to ensure the processes ran as smoothly as possible.

> My problem is that I got home last week from the taxi (after the circle meeting) and I've never been out the house since cause I can't, I live in a bungalow, great, no problems but I can't even get out my drive because I've got a rotator, both rotator cuffs but this one is shattered and I can't push (wheelchair) up hills so my thing is that I'm locked at home all the time. (CM Participant 6, T3)

The participant here is discussing the impact his mobility and housing issues have on his daily life. The location of the house he currently resides in, combined with his confinement to a manual wheelchair which he is unable to operate, means the CoSA sessions are the only time he leaves his house each week. As is reported within the literature, social isolation such as this, works against those convicted of sexual offences reintegrating successfully back into the community (Tewksbury & Mustaine, 2009). However, it can be argued that CoSA are going some way to prevent complete isolation from society, as without the weekly CoSA sessions the Core Member may not have interacted with outside civilisation at all.

The third issue concerning participants once released from prison was their continuous anxiety and worry of the public's opinions of them.

> Because of the nature of my crime, I'm very nervous about meeting new people, going out on my own anywhere and when I'm on the tram they've got some of those disabled seats, so I'm sitting side wards and you know people behind me, I'm very nervous of it, even on the bus I sit on the sideways seats, I'm always looking out but meeting new people on the group (CoSA) as I have done it's slowly bringing me out of that sort of stage so I'm venturing out a bit more and not so much trusting people but just getting out and about. (CM Participant 2, T3)

In the first half of the extract participant 2 is talking about a perceived threat of physical violence he constantly experiences when out in the community, which creates feelings of anxiety. The Core Member's fears are not unfounded due to the media's representation of those who commit sexual offences as sexual predators who should be hated and loathed (McAlinden, 2006). Although acts of violence towards those convicted of sexual offences are relatively uncommon (Tewksbury & Lees, 2006), the Core Members still have to deal with the fear of this stigmatisation. Being a Core Member on CoSA however, means they do not have to face it alone. In the second part of the extract, the Core Member is explaining how being part of CoSA has encouraged him to 'venture out' in the community more. Although he admits his trust of others has not increased, he is striving not to isolate himself.

> I suppose I'm under, I feel under pressure, I feel that I'm an outsider I suppose in how I feel…I don't feel that I'm relaxed, I can't relax, I don't know how…I feel I've lost my place like in the community. (Participant 6, T3)

Here the Core Member is describing how he now construes himself as an outsider in his old community with the new 'sex offender' identity overruling any previous identities. This is not uncommon for those who have committed sexual offences. For example, Mingus and Burchfield (2012) reported from their research with those who commit sexual offences that the 'sex offender' label is the most highly stigmatised label in modern societies such as the UK. They argued that the 'sex offender' status often becomes the master status above all other identities the person may have, such as a father or, in the case of this Core Member, a respected member of the local community. Within the literature, an internalisation of this stigmatisation towards ex-offenders is thought to predict both reconviction and re-imprisonment, even after controlling for the social problems they would face on re-entry in to the community (LeBel, Burnett, Maruna, & Bushway, 2008). Although LeBel et al's. (2008) research involved offenders convicted of all offence types, it still provides concerning findings for those who have previously committed sexual offences but are attempting to now live a crime-free life in the community.

Despite this fear of stigmatisation some of the Core Members describe how being part of CoSA has encouraged them to open up emotionally to other people.

> Circles helped as well but just realising that I needed to be able to talk more or to be more open with people cause I used to kind of like there was a brick wall round me and when anybody got too close I would just, whatever I needed to send them away I'd do it. (CM Participant 10, T3)

For this core member specifically, this is the first time they have ever taken the step to lower their emotional barriers, and being part of CoSA enables him to practice this before their Circle ends. This resonates with research on UK and Dutch CoSA, whereby Core Members developed their openness to communication within the CoSA, which lead to a positive ripple effect in the quality of their relationships outside the CoSA (Höing, Bogaerts, & Vogelvang, 2013). Improving the psychological wellbeing is an important aspect of CoSA's success that should not be overlooked when considering the effectiveness of CoSA projects (see Chap. 3 for more discussion on this). Offering support in this way, to help the Core Members develop new social bonds with the wider community is reported to help counteract any feelings of disconnectedness that may be felt through perceived stigmatisation from society (McNeill, 2009). In addition, encouraging the Core Members to overcome potential social isolation and loneliness by forming relations with others will hopefully help to lower their risk of reoffending (Marshall, 2010). What is unclear however, is whether this, along with the additional benefits described previously, is enough to enable desistance to truly take place.

General Discussion

From the research findings discussed, it can be argued that being part of a prison-based model CoSA enables individuals to receive pro-social support from a network of non-professionals, that they would otherwise be without. The additional prison sessions, allowed time for relationships between the Core Member and volunteers to be built and therefore extra support to be provided before the point of release. The benefit of this, in addition to improving the Core Members' wellbeing, is that individuals who have committed offences are more likely to accept specific guidance regarding desistance from individuals they have already established a relationship with (McCulloch, 2005).

Another benefit highlighted in the data was the role the additional prison sessions played in enabling the Core Member to be as prepared as possible for release. This was with regard specifically to the restrictions involved in their licence conditions and some of the possible risky situations they may find themselves in, all of which encouraged the Core Member to be accountable for their thoughts and behaviours. It is important to note here that whilst some Core Members felt comfortable in discussing the details of their sex offender treatment experiences, including any strategies they had developed to prevent reoffending in the future, this is not a necessary requirement. The sessions involved in CoSA of any type are unique and specific to the needs of the individual Core Members, and are not intended to replace sex offender treatment programmes in any way (Bates et al., 2014). In fact, Ward and Langlands (2009) warn against trying to combine or blend restorative justice practices such as CoSA with rehabilitative treatment, due them being complimentary but very different components of crime reduction, designed to deal with different tasks.

With regard to the Core Members' release from prison, being part of a prison-based model CoSA enabled support to be provided by the volunteers immediately on re-entry into community. This not only reduces anxiety for the Core Member, but also helps prevent them slipping back into old offending behaviour, during this heightened period of risk (Aresti et al., 2010). In addition, the CoSA sessions once in the community encouraged the Core Members to integrate with society, something they may not partake in otherwise due to health issues and the perceived stigmatisation of those around them.

Whilst the benefits to the additional sessions in the prison-based model have been documented, it is not clear whether these are in fact enough to ensure that desistance from crime is reached. As has been stated at several points throughout the chapter and argued in much more detail elsewhere (Graffam, Shinkfield, Lavelle, & McPherson, 2004; Tewksbury & Copes, 2013; Tewksbury & Mustaine, 2009), those who are convicted of a sexual offence face many barriers to successful reintegration. As LeBel et al. (2008) have reported, social problems experienced after release from prison, such as employment, housing and relationship issues, have a large and significant impact on the probability of both reconviction and re-imprisonment. Further research is therefore required in order to determine whether the benefits of the additional prison sessions in this new model of CoSA were sufficient enough to enable the Core Member to overcome the barriers to reintegration and reintegrate successfully back into the community. Returning to the Core Members once their time with the prison-based model of CoSA had ended would enable the true effectiveness of the model to be considered, with regard to how successful they had been in becoming a pro-social, active member of the community.

In conclusion, the findings suggest that a prison-based model of CoSA provides additional support to Core Members during their transition from prison to the community. Relationships can be established prior to release from prison, ensuring the CoSA 'hits the ground running' when reaching the community. In addition, preparing them for life as an ex-offender previously convicted of a sexual offence, ensures they are held accountable for their thoughts and behaviour. Further research is now required in order to establish how effective the benefits of a prison-based model of CoSA are in enabling individuals to overcome the barriers to successful reintegration.

References

Aresti, A., Eatough, V., & Brooks-Gordon, B. (2010). Doing time after time: An interpretative phenomenological analysis of reformed ex-offenders' experiences of self-change, identity and career opportunities. *Psychology, Crime & Law, 16*(3), 169–190. https://doi.org/10.1080/10683160802516273

Armstrong, S., Chistyakova, Y., Mackenzie, S., & Malloch, M. (2008). *Circles of support and accountability: Consideration of the feasibility of pilots in Scotland*. Commissioned report by the Scottish government. Glasgow: SCCJR. Retrieved from www.sccjr.ac.uk

Barnett, G. D., Wakeling, H. C., & Howard, P. D. (2010). An examination of the predictive validity of the risk matrix 2000 in England and Wales. *Sexual Abuse: A Journal of Research and Treatment, 22*(4), 443–470. https://doi.org/10.1177/1079063210384274

Barry, M. (2007). Listening and learning: The reciprocal relationship between worker and client. *Probation Journal, 54*(4), 407–422. https://doi.org/10.1177/0264550507083539

Bates, A., Williams, D., Wilson, C., & Wilson, R. J. (2014). Circles south east: The first 10 years 2002–2012. *International Journal of Offender Therapy and Comparative Criminology, 58*(7), 861–885. https://doi.org/10.1177/0306624X13485362

Berg, M. T., & Huebner, B. M. (2011). Re-entry and the ties that bind: An examination of social ties, employment, and recidivism. *Justice Quarterly, 28*(2), 382–410. https://doi.org/10.1080/07418825.2010.498383

Blagden, N., Winder, B., & Hames, C. (2016). "They treat us like human beings"—Experiencing a therapeutic sex offenders prison: Impact on offenders and staff and implications for treatment. *International Journal of Offender Therapy and Comparative Criminology, 60*(4), 371–396.

Bows, H., & Westmarland, N. (2016). Older sex offenders—Managing risk in the community from a policing perspective. *Policing and Society*, 1–13. https://doi.org/10.1080/10439463.2016.1138476

Brocki, J. M., & Wearden, A. J. (2006). A critical evaluation of the use of interpretative phenomenological analysis (IPA) in health psychology. *Psychology and Health, 21*(1), 87–108. https://doi.org/10.1080/14768320500230185

Clarke, M., Brown, S., & Völlm, B. (2015). Circles of support and accountability for sex offenders: A systematic review of outcomes. *Sexual Abuse: A Journal of Research and Treatment*, 1–33. https://doi.org/10.1177/1079063215603691

Craig, L. A., & Hutchinson, R. B. (2005). Sexual offenders with learning disabilities: Risk, recidivism and treatment. *Journal of Sexual Aggression, 11*(3), 289–304. https://doi.org/10.1080/13552600500273919

Crawley, E., & Sparks, R. (2005). Hidden injuries? Researching the experiences of older men in English prisons. *Howard Journal of Criminal Justice, 44*(4), 345–356. https://doi.org/10.1111/j.1468-2311.2005.00380.x

Crawley, E., & Sparks, R. (2006). Is there life after imprisonment? How elderly men talk about imprisonment and release. *Criminology and Criminal Justice, 6*(1), 63–82. https://doi.org/10.1177/1748895806060667

Cummins, R. A., & Lau, A. L. (2003). Community integration or community exposure? A review and discussion in relation to people with an intellectual disability. *Journal of Applied Research in Intellectual Disabilities, 16*(2), 145–157. https://doi.org/10.1046/j.1468-3148.2003.00157.x

Duwe, G. (2012). Can circles of support and accountability (COSA) work in the United States? Preliminary results from a randomized experiment in Minnesota. *Sexual Abuse: A Journal of Research and Treatment, 25*(2), 143–165. https://doi.org/10.1177/1079063212453942

Elliott, I. A., & Zajac, G. (2015). The implementation of circles of support and accountability in the United States. *Aggression and Violent Behavior, 25*, 113–123. https://doi.org/10.1016/j.avb.2015.07.014

Fazel, S., Sjöstedt, G., Långström, N., & Grann, M. (2006). Risk factors for criminal recidivism in older sexual offenders. *Sexual Abuse: A Journal of Research and Treatment, 18*(2), 159–167. https://doi.org/10.1177/107906320601800204

Fox, K. J. (2015). Contextualizing the policy and pragmatics of reintegrating sex offenders. *Sexual Abuse: A Journal of Research and Treatment*, 1–23. https://doi.org/10.1177/1079063215574711

Göbbels, S., Ward, T., & Willis, G. M. (2012). An integrative theory of desistance from sex offending. *Aggression and Violent Behavior, 17*(5), 453–462. https://doi.org/10.1016/j.avb.2012.06.003

Graffam, J., Shinkfield, A., Lavelle, B., & McPherson, W. (2004). Variables affecting successful reintegration as perceived by offenders and professionals. *Journal of Offender Rehabilitation, 40*(1–2), 147–171. https://doi.org/10.1300/j076v40n01_08

Hanson, R. K., & Morton-Bourgon, K. E. (2005). The characteristics of persistent sexual offenders: A meta-analysis of recidivism studies. *Journal of Consulting and Clinical Psychology, 73*(6), 1154–1163. https://doi.org/10.1037/0022-006X.73.6.1154

Hanvey, S., Philpot, T., & Wilson, C. (2011). *A community based approach to the reduction of sexual offending: Circles of Support and Accountability*. London: Jessica Kingsley Publishers.

Hart, M. (2008). The geriatric sex offender: Senile or paedophile. *Law & Psychology Review, 32*, 153–162.

Hayes, S., Shackell, P., Mottram, P., & Lancaster, R. (2007). The prevalence of intellectual disability in a major UK prison. *British Journal of Learning Disabilities, 35*(3), 162–167. https://doi.org/10.1111/j.1468-3156.2007.00461.x

Höing, M., Bogaerts, S., & Vogelvang, B. (2013). Circles of support and accountability: How and why they work for sex offenders. *Journal of Forensic Psychology Practice, 13*(4), 267–295. https://doi.org/10.1080/15228932.2013.808526

Höing, M., Vogelvang, B., & Bogaerts, S. (2015). "I am a different man now"-sex offenders in circles of support and accountability: A prospective study. *International Journal of Offender Therapy and Comparative Criminology*, 1–22. https://doi.org/10.1177/0306624x15612431

Howse, K. (2003). *Growing old in prison: A scoping study on older prisoners*. London, UK: Prison Reform Trust.

Ievins, A. (2013). *Living among sex offenders: Identity, safety and relationships at Whatton prison*. Masters dissertation, Cambridge University, UK.

King, S. (2013). Assisted desistance and experiences of probation supervision. *Probation Journal, 60*(2), 136–151. https://doi.org/10.1177/0264550513478320

Kitson-Boyce, R., Blagden, N., Winder, B., & Dillon, G. (2018a). *'This time it's different' preparing for release through CoSA (The prison model): A phenomenological and repertory grid analysis.* Manuscript submitted for publication.

Kitson-Boyce, R., Blagden, N., Winder, B., & Dillon, G. (2018b). *The need for a prison-based model of circles of support and accountability: Cognitive change and the shadow of release.* Manuscript submitted for publication.

Lambrick, F., & Glaser, W. (2004). Sex offenders with an intellectual disability. *Sexual Abuse: A Journal of Research and Treatment, 16*(4), 381–392. https://doi.org/10.1023/b:sebu.0000043330.65936.66

LeBel, T. P., Burnett, R., Maruna, S., & Bushway, S. (2008). The chicken and egg' of subjective and social factors in desistance from crime. *European Journal of Criminology, 5*(2), 131–159. https://doi.org/10.1177/1477370807087640

Levenson, J. S., Brannon, Y. N., Fortney, T., & Baker, J. (2007). Public perceptions about sex offenders and community protection policies. *Analyses of Social Issues and Public Policy, 7*(1), 137–161. https://doi.org/10.1111/j.1530-2415.2007.00119.x

Lindsay, W. (2002). Research and literature on sex offenders with intellectual and developmental disabilities. *Journal of Intellectual Disability Research, 46*(s1), 74–85. https://doi.org/10.1046/j.1365-2788.2002.00006.x

Lussier, P., & Gress, C. L. (2014). Community re-entry and the path toward desistance: A quasi-experimental longitudinal study of dynamic factors and community risk management of adult sex offenders. *Journal of Criminal Justice, 42*(2), 111–122. https://doi.org/10.1016/j.jcrimjus.2013.09.006

Maguire, M., & Raynor, P. (2006). How the resettlement of prisoners promotes desistance from crime or does it? *Criminology and Criminal Justice, 6*(1), 19–38. https://doi.org/10.1177/1748895806060665

Marshall, W. L. (2010). The role of attachments, intimacy, and loneliness in the etiology and maintenance of sexual offending. *Sexual and Relationship Therapy, 25*(1), 73–85. https://doi.org/10.1080/14681990903550191

Maruna, S. (2001). *Making good: How ex-convicts reform and rebuild their lives.* Washington, DC: American Psychological Association Books.

McAlinden, A. (2006). Managing risk from regulation to the reintegration of sexual offenders. *Criminology and Criminal Justice, 6*(2), 197–218. https://doi.org/10.1177/1748895806062981

McCartan, K. (2015, October). *Circles of support and accountability in the UK.* Paper presented at the Association of the Treatment of Sexual Abusers 34th Annual Research and Treatment Conference, Montreal, QC, Canada.

McCartan, K., Kemshall, H., Westwood, S., Solle, J., MacKenzie, G., & Pollard, A. (2014). *Circles of Support and Accountability (CoSA): A case file review of two pilots*. Ministry of Justice Analytical Summary. London: Ministry of Justice.

McCulloch, T. (2005). Probation, social context and desistance: Retracing the relationship. *Probation Journal, 52*(1), 8–22. https://doi.org/10.1177/0264550505050623

McNeill, F. (2009). What works and what's just? *European Journal of Probation, 1*(1), 21–40. https://doi.org/10.1177/206622030900100103

McNeill, F., & Weaver, E. (2010). *Changing lives? Desistance research and offender management*. Report No. 03/2010. Scotland: The Scottish Centre for Crime and Justice Research.

Mingus, W., & Burchfield, K. B. (2012). From prison to integration: Applying modified labelling theory to sex offenders. *Criminal Justice Studies, 25*(1), 97–109. https://doi.org/10.1080/1478601X.2012.657906

MnCoSA. (2017). MnCoSA Circle Member. *Idealist*. Retrieved from https://www.idealist.org/en/volunter-opportunity/f0e705fe443b45d9a8411460d65e4107-mncosa-circle-member-mncosa-saint-paul

Nellis, M. (2009). Circles of support and accountability for sex offenders in England and Wales: Their origins and implementation between 1999–2005. *British Journal of Community Justice, 7*(1), 22–44. https://doi.org/10.1080/10282580701372046

Northcutt Bohmert, M. N., Duwe, G., & Hipple, N. K. (2016). Evaluating restorative justice circles of support and accountability can social support overcome structural barriers? *International Journal of Offender Therapy and Comparative Criminology*, 1–20. https://doi.org/10.1177/0306624X16652627

Pratt, D., Piper, M., Appleby, L., Webb, R., & Shaw, J. (2006). Suicide in recently released offenders: A population-based cohort study. *The Lancet, 368*(9530), 119–123. https://doi.org/10.1016/S0140-6736(06)69002-8

Rocque, M., Bierie, D. M., & MacKenzie, D. L. (2011). Social bonds and change during incarceration: Testing a missing link in the re-entry research. *International Journal of Offender Therapy and Comparative Criminology, 55*(5), 816–838. https://doi.org/10.1177/0306624x10370457

Schwaebe, C. (2005). Learning to pass: Sex offenders' strategies for establishing a viable identity in the prison general population. *International Journal of Offender Therapy and Comparative Criminology, 49*(6), 614–625. https://doi.org/10.1177/0306624x05275829

Serin, R. C., & Lloyd, C. D. (2009). Examining the process of offender change: The transition to crime desistance. *Psychology, Crime & Law, 15*(4), 347–364. https://doi.org/10.1080/10683160802261078

Shaw, J. A., & Budd, E. C. (1982). Determinants of acquiescence and naysaying of mentally retarded persons. *American Journal of Mental Deficiency, 87*, 108–110.

Smith, J. A., & Osborn, M. (2003). Interpretative phenomenological analysis. In J. A. Smith (Ed.), *Qualitative psychology: A practical guide to research methods* (pp. 51–80). London: Sage.

Tewksbury, R. (2012). Stigmatization of sex offenders. *Deviant Behavior, 33*(8), 606–623. https://doi.org/10.1080/01639625.2011.636690

Tewksbury, R., & Connor, D. P. (2012). Incarcerated sex offenders' perceptions of family relationships: Previous experiences and future expectations. *Western Criminology Review, 13*(2), 25–35. https://doi.org/10.1177/0032885512467318

Tewksbury, R., & Copes, H. (2013). Incarcerated sex offenders' expectations for re-entry. *The Prison Journal, 93*(1), 102–122. https://doi.org/10.1177/0032885512467318

Tewksbury, R., & Lees, M. (2006). Perceptions of sex offender registration: Collateral consequences and community experiences. *Sociological Spectrum, 26*(3), 309–334. https://doi.org/10.1080/02732170500524246

Tewksbury, R., & Mustaine, E. E. (2009). Stress and collateral consequences for registered sex offenders. *Journal of Public Management & Social Policy, 15*(2), 215–239.

Thomas, T., Thompson, D., & Karstedt. (2014). *Assessing the impact of Circles of Support and Accountability on the reintegration of adults convicted of sexual offences in the community*. Leeds: Centre for Criminal Justice Studies, University of Leeds.

Thornton, D., Mann, R., Webster, S., Blud, L., Travers, R., Friendship, C., et al. (2003). Distinguishing and combining risks for sexual and violent recidivism. *Annals of the New York Academy of Sciences, 989*(1), 225–235. https://doi.org/10.1111/j.1749-6632.2003.tb07308.x

Van den Berg, C., Beijersbergen, K., Nieuwbeerta, P., & Dirkzwager, A. (2017). Sex offenders in prison: Are they socially isolated? *Sexual Abuse*, 1–18. https://doi.org/10.1177/1079063217700884

Ward, T., & Langlands, R. (2009). Repairing the rupture: Restorative justice and the rehabilitation of offenders. *Aggression and Violent Behavior, 14*(3), 205–214. https://doi.org/10.1016/j.avb.2009.03.001

Weaver, B., & McNeill, F. (2015). Lifelines desistance, social relations, and reciprocity. *Criminal Justice and Behavior, 42*(1), 95–107. https://doi.org/10.1177/0093854814550031

Willis, G. M., & Grace, R. C. (2008). The quality of community reintegration planning for child molesters: Effects on sexual recidivism. *Sexual Abuse: A Journal of Research and Treatment, 20*(2), 218–240. https://doi.org/10.1177/1079063208318005

Wilson, C., Bates, A., & Völlm, B. (2010). Circles of support and accountability: An innovative approach to manage high-risk sex offenders in the community. *Open Criminology Journal, 3*, 48–57. https://doi.org/10.2174/1874917801003010048

Wilson, R. J., Picheca, J. E., & Prinzo, M. (2005). *Circles of support and accountability: An evaluation of the pilot project in South-Central Ontario*. Ottawa, ON: Correctional Service of Canada.

5

Evaluating Community-Based Circles of Support and Accountability

Michelle Dwerryhouse

Introduction

Evaluation research is used to assess the quality and impact of a social intervention; it is important to ensure that an intervention is being carried out to the best possible standards, highlighting areas of improvement and assessing if the intervention makes a difference (or not) and to whom. Evaluation research also demonstrates the success of a social intervention (Moore et al., 2015). A good evaluation should encompass all stakeholders in order to gain a complete picture of the intervention. An intervention may appear to be successful on the surface, yet hold flaws unknown to all parties. A service provider may perceive an intervention to be successful, whilst a service user may experience a poor intervention which they perceive to be unsuccessful. If an evaluation only takes account of one party's views, the subsequent findings would not provide a true picture.

M. Dwerryhouse (✉)
Nottingham Trent University, Nottingham, UK

H. Elliott et al. (eds.), *Sexual Crime and Circles of Support and Accountability*, Sexual Crime, https://doi.org/10.1007/978-3-319-74823-8_5

Where possible it is beneficial to carry out a process evaluation rather than evaluating an intervention retrospectively. Process evaluations begin during implementation and determine whether the intervention is operating as planned. This allows for adjustments to be made as and when required for the improvement of the intervention (Moore et al., 2015). In some cases is it not possible or suitable to carry out a process evaluation, in which case an outcome evaluation may be chosen. Outcome evaluations are used to measure the effectiveness of the intervention and to determine how well the goals of the intervention have been achieved.

Evaluation outcomes may be positive or negative and are unique to the evaluation being carried out. Taking Circles of Support and Accountability (CoSA) as an example, positive outcomes may include desistance promotion; improved emotional wellbeing of Core Members; increases in Core Members social network; attainment of permanent accommodation and employment opportunities. Alternatively, a negative outcome may present as the Core Member reoffending. Evaluation outcomes may cover both emotional elements such as changes in Core Member self-esteem and happiness and practical elements such as changes in Core Member employment and accommodation. All outcomes, both positive and negative should be used as a tool from which to learn and improve practice.

The topics discussed in this chapter cover important areas of research which should be considered in an evaluation of CoSA comprising both process and outcome. In order to obtain the most from evaluation, research methods must be selected carefully and appropriately according to the area of interest. It is proposed that mixed methods are both suitable and necessary for a full evaluation of CoSA. The topics covered are Core Member risk of recidivism; Core Member emotional wellbeing; success and failure in CoSA and consideration of the volunteers and professionals involved with CoSA.

Part 1: Understanding Changes in Core Members and Risk of Reoffending

Recidivism rates for individuals convicted of sexual offences are highest during the first few years following release (Hanson, Harris, Helmus, & Thornton, 2014). The recidivism rate reduces from 22% to 8.6% for those who desist from reoffending for five years following release from prison and reduces further to 4.2% at ten years post release (Hanson et al., 2014). Whilst in prison and upon release, individuals convicted of sexual offences are subject to risk assessments, used to determine the level of risk they pose to others, both in the short and long term (Beech, Fisher, & Thornton, 2003). There are both static and dynamic risk assessments, which assess fixed and changeable factors relating to risk respectively. Experience of an abusive childhood, low intelligence and prior offences are examples of static risk factors. They have been shown to influence risk, but are not open to intervention and are therefore classed as static or unchangeable, although it is important to note they can change over time, for example a person's offending history can increase (Andrews & Bonta, 2010; Mann, Hanson, & Thornton, 2010). Alternatively, dynamic risk refers to changeable factors which are amenable to intervention. Poor relationships with friends and family, substance misuse and offence related attitudes are examples of dynamic risk factors (Andrews & Bonta, 2010).

Within the prison setting many individuals convicted of a sexual offence are assessed using a dynamic risk assessment called the Structured Assessment of Risk and Need (SARN; Thornton, 2002), which formed the basis for the development of the CoSA Dynamic Risk Review (DRR). Developed and introduced by Circles UK in 2009, the DRR is a tool created to assess Core Members' dynamic risk over time whilst engaging with CoSA. It is based upon the four dynamic risk domains identified within the SARN: sexual interests; offence related attitudes; relationships and self-management. The DRR was designed to be used at the start of CoSA and again at three monthly intervals throughout the course of the CoSA. This allows for overall dynamic risk to be measured over time as well as enabling monitoring of specific risk domains. The ability to measure changes within risk domains has the potential to be used by the CoSA to inform interventions specific to individual Core Members and their needs.

Core Member Dynamic Risk in the Community

Bates and Wager (2016) assessed adverse outcomes following completion of CoSA, by assessing thirteen Core Members' DRRs (where a minimum of three were completed per Core Member). Adverse outcomes were noted as inappropriate or illegal behavior by the Core Member such as arrest, recall to prison, reconviction or breach of license. However, it is important to note that reconviction may have related to historical offences pre-dating the CoSA. Thirteen Core Members with adverse endings were compared against a matched control group of Core Members with no adverse outcomes. Controls were matched on the basis that they came from the same CoSA project and had the same number of completed DRRs. Age was also matched as closely as possible, although due to numbers this was not always possible. The results of the study indicated a statistically significant reduction in DRR scores over time in the matched control group, demonstrating a reduction in dynamic risk. In comparison Core Members in the adverse outcome group did not show such a decline. This research provides evidence for the effectiveness of the DRR in predicting the adverse outcomes noted (which includes its ability to predict reconviction). Additionally the predictive ability of the DRR can be used to highlight specific Core Members who may present an increased recidivism risk. In the United Kingdom, many individuals are managed in the community by Offender Managers who work within the National Probation Service. Information contained in the DRR is valuable for Offender Managers who may choose to increase surveillance. It can also be used in conjunction with other aspects of CoSA evaluation research to pinpoint areas for improvement. One such area is that of success and failure in CoSA which is discussed in Part 3. Table 5.1 below details the risk domains of the DRR, along with examples of how each domain can be utilised in supporting the rehabilitation of the Core Member.

An evaluation of CoSA is an opportunity to evaluate both the process of regular assessments and the outcomes of those assessments; in this case, changes in Core Members' dynamic risk over time. Whilst poor procedural processes may weaken the ability to evaluate risk outcomes, it does provide an opportunity to improve data collection processes. An evaluation carried out over a longitudinal period would allow time for processes to be tightened and subsequent outcome data to be most reliable. The same considerations should also be given to data concerning Core Members' emotional wellbeing, discussed next.

Table 5.1 Dynamic risk domains

Domain	Explanation
A Sexual interests	Within a CoSA, Core Members are encouraged to speak openly about any sexual thoughts they may have. It is the role of the volunteers to challenge any inappropriate thoughts that the Core Member may present whilst offering a safe place for Core Members to discuss their thoughts and feelings.
B Offence related attitudes	As with domain A, Core Members are given the opportunity to discuss their attitudes with the CoSA and are challenged on any inappropriate attitudes. Furthermore, CoSA volunteers are usually designed to contain a mix of males and females. This is especially important in cases whereby, for example, the Core Member has specific issues concerning females. The presence of both males and females working together and supporting each other positively demonstrates male—female relationships. This is something which is also practiced within the prison setting for treatment programmes.
C Relationships	The CoSA exists to support rehabilitation and integration and hold the Core Member accountable for their actions. Core Members may feel that they are inadequate and undeserving of a relationship. They may also experience low self-esteem relating to their perceived capabilities in relation to employment. This is an example of where the support function comes into play. Volunteers can help to support Core Members to build their self-esteem and sense of self-worth through activities. CoSA is about more than talking through thoughts and feelings; volunteers help to support the Core Member to pursue meaningful activities such as employment, voluntary work and hobbies.
	Volunteers also assist Core Members to meet new people and make friends and even support Core Members in building new and appropriate romantic relationships. There are endless opportunities for Core Members to gain confidence and increase self-esteem, which in turn is expected to reduce dynamic risk. Moreover, volunteers continuing support for Core Members instils a belief in Core Members that they have the ability to change and to lead a positive offence free life. This has the ability to encourage Core Members to desist from offending (Fox, 2016).

(*continued*)

Table 5.1 (continued)

Domain	Explanation
D Self-management	There may be occasions when a Core Member is faced with a risky situation. Within a CoSA, the Core Member is offered the opportunity to discuss and reflect upon such situations. Together the CoSA can devise tactics for dealing with difficult situations, such as crossing the road if an attractive person is walking towards them in the street, or avoiding being outside during school opening and closing times. In doing this, Core Members are encouraged to proactively prepare for situations which may put them at risk of reoffending and act to discourage impulsive behaviour.

Part 2: Understanding Changes in Core Member Emotional Wellbeing over Time

Individuals convicted of a sexual offence are surrounded by stigma. Upon release from prison, individuals convicted of sexual offences are subject to sexual offence registry laws. This means that an individual is tainted by the 'sex offender' label permanently. The label serves as a life sentence, regardless of whether the individual reoffends or not. If the same individual had instead committed another serious offence such as murder, they would not be subject to such labels of permanence. Sexual offences hold something of a taboo within society that other serious offences do not (Mingus & Burchfield, 2012).

Breakdowns in relationships and rifts between friendships can happen to anyone. Although for people who have committed sexual offences, it is common for mass disownment to take place. It is often difficult for friends and family to accept such offences were perpetrated by their loved one. On other occasions friends and family may wish to avoid the stigma of being associated with such an individual for fear they themselves will be vilified (Bailey & Sample, 2017). Research has reported how some individuals deny their offences to friends and family for fear of losing contact (Blagden, Winder, Thorne, & Gregson, 2011). Schmitt, Branscombe, Postmes, and Garcia (2014) carried out a meta-analysis into the effect of stigma upon emotional wellbeing. The findings evidenced the strong negative impact of stigma upon the perceiver's emotional wellbeing including items such as depression, anxiety and self-esteem. Although individuals convicted of sexual offences were not included in the analysis, it is argued that they would experience negative effects to a similar, if not greater extent due to being amongst the most stigmatised individuals in society. Additionally such stigma in the community may contribute towards initiating a self-fulfilling prophecy in the individual whereby the individual begins to believe in the risk they have come to be associated with and so acts out in congruence with such behaviours (Schultz, 2014).

Furthermore, Core Members encounter prejudice on a daily basis when faced with media portrayals that sensationalise sexual crime in an attempt to increase sales, with sexual crimes being nine times over-represented when compared to national crime statistics (Harper & Hogue, 2015). Media portrayals also lead ex-offenders to become isolated from their community, which further increases risk (Malinen, Willis, & Johnston, 2014). Such labelling can make it difficult for some individuals to move on, inhibiting their ability to create a new identity for themselves in which they are no longer identified as a 'sex offender'. Regardless of their histories, such individuals are people who have much to contribute to society if given the opportunity. However, whilst surrounded by stigma, an individual is not afforded the opportunity to reach their pro-social potential. This is illustrated in Maslow's hierarchy of needs (Maslow, 1943) whereby each tier is argued to be unobtainable without first meeting the needs of the lower tier (Fig. 5.1).

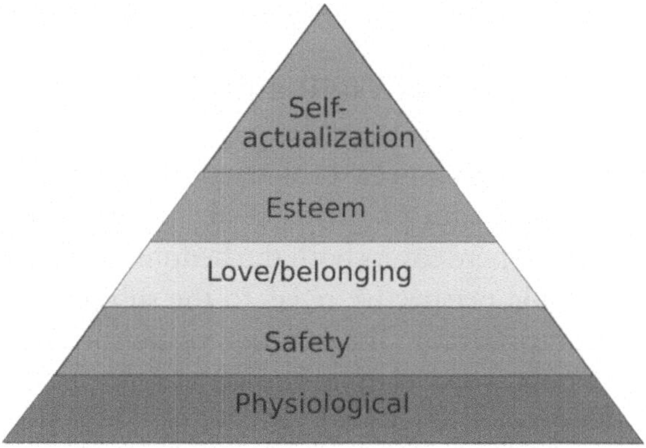

Fig. 5.1 Representation of Maslow's hierarchy of needs

The average person has a support network surrounding them; friends, family, partners, work colleagues. Think about the people in your life. Now, take a minute to imagine if everyone you knew suddenly chose to disregard or abandon you. Imagine a version of your life in which every single person who conversed with you only did so because they were paid to. It's a difficult thing to imagine. It's an even more difficult thing to live with. Yet this is what many ex-offenders have to live with on a day to day basis, often for months or years on end. CoSA offers the opportunity to escape such isolation, if only for one or two hours each week. For someone who has nobody, that can mean a lot.

The impact of this label and the media representation is discussed in detail in Chap. 6. It is expected that participation in CoSA has the potential to improve Core Members emotional wellbeing by providing a supportive environment in which Core Members are treated respectfully, as equals, and are not subject to stigma or prejudice. The CoSA allows the Core Member the time and space to feel comfortable opening up and discussing their offence and their feelings about their perceived ongoing risk without fear of persecution.

The knowledge that CoSA are made up of community volunteers who give their time freely and willingly is in itself a major benefit to the Core Member. Many do not have any support structures in place outside of the professionals they must meet with. The simple fact that the Core Member has four to six people who are not paid to be there can go a long way in improving a Core Member's emotional wellbeing.

Core Member Emotional Wellbeing in the Community

Mental wellbeing refers to aspects of our emotions which serve to promote positive mental health (Tennant et al., 2007). The definition of mental wellbeing used here covers both the hedonic and eudaimonic perspectives. The hedonic perspective refers to the subjective experience of happiness and life satisfaction. The eudaimonic perspective refers to psychological functioning, good relationships with others and self-realisation. The eudaimonic perspective covers a wide range of cognitive aspects of mental health (Tennant et al., 2007). See Ryan and Deci (2001) for an in-depth explanation. The eudaimonic perspective includes aspects related to emotional and physical wellbeing (Ryan & Deci, 2001), therefore the terms emotional and mental wellbeing will be used interchangeably.

Some examples of positive cognitive aspects of emotional wellbeing are high self-esteem, internal locus of control and strong coping skills. Many Core Members are deficient in these when they first join CoSA, and such deficiencies can often contribute toward risk of harm. The following examples illustrate this, and explain how the presence of CoSA can assist to promote positive change in Core Members' emotional wellbeing.

Low Self Esteem

Self-esteem is defined by how much value people place on themselves, and their perception of their self-worth (Baumeister, Campbell, Krueger, & Vohs, 2003). High self-esteem has been linked with increased happiness whilst low self-esteem has been linked to depression (Baumeister et al., 2003). Individuals convicted of sexual offences may have low self-esteem due to the negative bias they are subjected to on a daily basis (Harper & Hogue, 2015). An ex-offender who has low self-esteem may not have the confidence or self-belief to apply for a job or attend an interview. In severe cases, low self-esteem may discourage an ex-offender from interacting with others in the community, which may contribute to poor social skills. This in turn could have repercussions for ex-offenders' isolation. Social isolation is among one of the most widely accepted risk factors for recidivism (Malinen et al., 2014). Through participation in CoSA, Core Members can be supported through the process of applying for work. This is particularly important and useful for those Core Members who have difficulty with their literacy and numeracy skills. Volunteers can also help Core Members with poor social skills, for example through role playing social scenarios and with confidence building by accompanying Core Members on trips to the shops or to social activities and hobbies.

External Locus of Control

Locus of Control (LOC) was developed by Rotter (1966) and refers to how an individual believes their life and life events to be within their control or controlled by external forces such as fate. LOC is described as being either internal (I control what happens in my life) or external (Fate/Destiny controls what happens in my life). LOC is important in mental health because external LOC has been linked to poorer health outcomes such as depression (Sullivan, Thompson, Kounali, Lewis, & Zammit, 2017). Research into sexual offences and LOC has reported that individuals with an external LOC tend to be those who carry out contact offences rather than internet offences. Moreover, individuals who carry out contact offences hold significantly more cognitive distortions about children such as beliefs that the child did not come to harm during sexual abuse, than individuals who carry out internet offences (Elliott, Beech, Mandeville-Norden, & Hayes, 2009). An ex-offender with an external locus of control may believe that their sexually abusive behaviour towards others is out of their control. They may hold the belief that their behaviour is inevitable, that it is an integral part of them and will happen regardless of any efforts made to the contrary. If an ex-offender believes that their sexually abusive behaviour is out of their control, their risk of recidivism is increased (McAnena, Craissati, & Southgate, 2016). Because an external LOC is associated with cognitive distortions it can be a difficult area for volunteers to tackle. However with the support of volunteers, Core Members can learn to take accountability for their own behaviour and come to realise that they have control over their own actions. This can be done through CoSA discussions. Research by (Höing, Vogelvang, & Bogaerts, 2015) has also reported how Core Members found their CoSA useful for exploring their cognitions in a safe environment, where they could rely on volunteers to advise and guide them, with some Core Members stating that participating in CoSA taught them to take different viewpoints in relation to their offence, including that of their victim.

Poor Coping Skills

Pearlin and Schooler (1978) refer to coping as things that people do to avoid being harmed by life-strains. Some individuals convicted of sexual offences use sex as a coping mechanism to deal with life-strains (Hanson & Hanson, 2007). Other individuals with poor coping skills may use drugs or alcohol to cope with their problems. This poses a risk toward both the health of the ex-offender and to others in the community due to the inhibition loss associated with such substances. With the support of CoSA, Core Members can learn to replace substance abuse with more therapeutic activities in order to cope with day to day difficulties, such as exercising or spending time on a hobby. Improvements in coping skills are linked to improvements in problem solving skills, a protective factor in the promotion of desistance (de Vries Robbé, Mann, Maruna, & Thornton, 2015).

The above are examples of some of the many factors which can influence emotional wellbeing. As illustrated, CoSA can provide support for a Core Member in a number of areas where they may otherwise have none. Through inclusion in CoSA, the ex-offender becomes the Core Member. This new label immediately allows the Core Member to take on a positive identity. The Core Member is viewed as a brave individual, willing to openly discuss their offence history. In making this difficult decision to seek support with a group of strangers, the Core Member actively chooses to take accountability for their previous offending behaviour in an attempt to build a new life. Whilst treatment programmes completed in prison are often mandatory, CoSA is entered into voluntarily. Therefore, it may be argued that by choosing to join CoSA, Core Members are actively pursuing a positive future, free from offending. Through inclusion in CoSA, the Core Member is no longer left alone to deal with the difficulties they may face on a daily basis. Instead, the Core Member has a support network of people promoting positive behaviour and assisting with their reintegration.

The Warwick-Edinburgh Mental Well-Being Scale (WEMWBS; Tennant et al., 2007) is a scale used to measure mental wellbeing through the use of 14 positively worded items. Although the WEMWBS has not been used with Core Members previously, it has been validated for use with both student and population samples in England and Scotland (Tennant et al., 2007). The WEMWBS is suitable for use on a forensic population as the statements used within the tool are generic on a human level so they apply to everyone, regardless of background. Research using the WEMWBS would enable the effectiveness of CoSA upon Core Member emotional wellbeing to be evaluated throughout the term of the CoSA.

Similar to the DRR discussed in Part 1, the WEMWBS has a number of practical uses. If the CoSA has a positive impact upon Core Members emotional wellbeing, we would expect to see improvements in WEMWBS scores over time. Secondly, comparisons can be made between Core Member emotional wellbeing and population norms on a large scale, whilst also providing the opportunity to identify individuals with particularly poor emotional wellbeing. This allows for targeted interventions to be aimed at the most vulnerable Core Members. Thirdly, wellbeing scores can be used in conjunction with DRR scores to increase understanding regarding the relationship between emotional wellbeing and dynamic risk. This triangulation of data could also be adopted in the following section exploring CoSA success and failure. This would aid understanding of how emotional wellbeing affects the relative success or failure of CoSA. It is expected that poor emotional wellbeing would be associated with CoSA failure, whilst Core Members with good or improved emotional wellbeing will be associated with successful CoSA outcomes.

Part 3: Success and Failure in CoSA

There are a number of benefits to be gained from CoSA continuing to its minimum term of twelve months, such as improvements in emotional wellbeing discussed in Part 2 (Clarke, Brown, & Völlm, 2015) and the accountability aspect which volunteers are encouraged to cover in CoSA discussions. Furthermore, reductions in recidivism are a potential, although yet unconfirmed benefit of successfully completed CoSA (Clarke et al., 2015). CoSA are designed to last between twelve to eighteen months, with volunteers and Core Members agreeing at the beginning of a Circle to commit to this time. However, for a number of reasons this is not always the case and some CoSA disband before the minimum twelve month term.

One way of beginning to explore attrition in CoSA is to consider the reasons for treatment attrition amongst individuals convicted of sexual offences. CoSA are not a treatment and should not be thought of as such (Bates, Williams, Wilson, & Wilson, 2013; Fox, 2015; Wilson, McWhinnie, & Wilson, 2008), however there are a number of similarities in the ways in which attrition occurs between the two interventions. Larochelle, Diguer, Laverdière, and Greenman (2011) evaluated the literature on treatment attrition and developed three main causes of treatment non-completion: premature termination by the offender; exclusion from treatment by the treatment team on the grounds of unacceptable behaviour or lack of participation; and termination of treatment due to recall to prison or a failure to comply with probation release conditions.

Factors Influencing CoSA Attrition

Although there is a paucity of research into unsuccessful CoSA, studies have noted a number of factors which lead to early unplanned CoSA endings, which can be broadly defined as Core Member dropout, recall to prison, Core Member exclusion or volunteer disbandment (Bates et al., 2013; Höing et al., 2015). Previously, Core Members have cited reasons for their voluntary withdrawal as a lack of motivation (Bates et al., 2013), a strong focus on accountability (Fox, 2015) and concerns over a lack of volunteer commitment or cooperation (Höing et al., 2015). In other cases, Core Members have been excluded from CoSA due to a lack of cooperation (Höing et al., 2015). There have also been occasions where Core Members have been recalled to prison for non-recent offences (Bates et al., 2013).

The idea that a strong focus on accountability can lead to early CoSA ending is an interesting one. McCartan (2016) noted how Core Members believed the CoSA existed to support rather than hold accountable, and research has evidenced that CoSA deemed to be the most successful are those in which the focus of discussion is around support rather than accountability (Fox, 2015). Moreover, Fox (2016) suggested that a minimisation of the accountability aspect may improve the desistance process for Core Members. These findings bring into question the value of the accountability aspect of CoSA and whether this aspect is in fact detrimental to Core Member reintegration. This is not to say that Core Members should not be held accountable for their historical offences. Rather it is suggested that CoSA may be more effective if they entail a future-focussed, strength based approach around protective factors, whilst acknowledging although not focussing, upon their ongoing risk. This would allow Core Members the opportunity to step away from an offender identity and develop an awareness of their positive attributes, whilst building their good life plan (Purvis, Ward, & Willis, 2011).

Research has shown that volunteering within CoSA can be a stressful task due to the intensive nature of work involved (Höing, Bogaerts, & Vogelvang, 2016). Because a lack of volunteer commitment has been cited as a reason for Core Member voluntary dropout, this holds implications for the selection and recruitment of suitable volunteers. Watson, Thomas, and Daffern (2015) noted how an offender's therapeutic environment can negatively affect offender outcomes. It could be argued that a positive therapeutic environment is equally important for Core Members receiving support through CoSA.

Beyko and Wong (2005) have argued that good therapeutic relationships can reduce offender dropout from treatment. It is argued that such negative effects may also be reversed through positive relationships. Many Core Members lack social support from friends and family and in the case of volunteer disbandment, such Core Members are likely to feel neglected and once again isolated. This in turn may have negative consequences for Core Member recidivism and integration. Research has evidenced that individuals who drop-out of treatment have higher rates of recidivism than treatment completers (Hanson et al., 2002). Furthermore, individuals who have had their treatment terminated early by a therapist have been evidenced to reoffend at a higher rate than those who drop-out from treatment (Swinburne Romine, Miner, Poplin, Dwyer, & Berg, 2012). If attrition rates in CoSA are similar to treatment attrition, there may be cause for concern over Core Members who choose to voluntarily withdraw from CoSA earlier than planned and cases whereby Core Members are left without a Circle due to volunteer disbandment.

In the absence of a theoretical construct of CoSA failure, it is argued that unsuccessful treatment interventions are used as a basis from which to understand unsuccessful CoSA. CoSA, much like the individuals that belong to them, vary in the rehabilitative approach taken. Whilst some CoSA end prematurely, others thrive. One factor which contributes to CoSA success is trusting and reciprocal relationships within the CoSA (Höing et al., 2016). As part of the accountability aspect of CoSA, Core Members are encouraged to discuss difficult topics with their volunteers relating to their own concerns about their risk. Core Members may be used to such discussions with the professionals in their lives but they also know that volunteers are different. Initially opening up to a group of strangers about their offence is no doubt a difficult task. Furthermore, Core Members are encouraged to continue such discussions about their accountability and any risk related thoughts that may occur on a weekly basis. For this reason, it is essential that Core Members feel they are in a comfortable environment, free from judgement, in which they can openly discuss their thoughts without fear of persecution. Some positive outcomes of CoSA involvement include a sense of social inclusion provided to Core Members which has been linked to improved self-esteem, support in transitions and skills such as problem solving behaviour, coping with emotions, self-care and social skills (Höing et al., 2016). However, such outcomes would not be possible without the presence of a supportive volunteer network. Therefore, it appears it is the supportive function of volunteers toward Core Members which has a positive influence on the eventual success of CoSA.

Part 4: The Experiences of Volunteers and Professionals in CoSA

Through interviews with CoSA volunteers, McCartan (2016) ascertained that volunteers felt CoSA was beneficial to the Core Members in terms of offering social and emotional support. The research also noted how seriously the volunteers took their role within the CoSA, as the volunteers were always aware of the importance of the role they had in the Core Member's risk management. The volunteers took their responsibilities seriously and were always cautious when choosing to report risky behaviour back to stakeholders, so as not to disrupt the supportive relationships which had been built with the Core Member. Furthermore, volunteers claimed to feel well supported and educated through the training they received when joining CoSA. Volunteers described themselves as pro-social role models and viewed the CoSA as a safe place in which the Core Member is free to discuss their views openly and without persecution (McCartan, 2016). However, the research reported that the volunteer's views of the CoSA were at odds with the Core Members behaviour; as volunteers often faced difficulties when attempting to encourage Core Members to engage in discussions around accountability. Whilst the Core Members were happy to be supported in many areas of their life, they were less forthcoming when faced with topics relating to their risk and potential for reoffending. This suggests that although Core Members are presented with a safe place to discuss their risk and accountability without judgement, they would rather spend the time discussing other topics.

In this sense, CoSA are viewed more in terms of its supportive function rather than that of accountability. As noted in Part 3, research has evidenced that the most successful CoSA are those in which the focus of discussion is around support rather than accountability (Fox, 2015). It could be argued that it is volunteer support which reduces recidivism, whereas an emphasis on Core Member accountability may have a negative effect in terms of further stigmatising the Core Member. Research into success and failure of CoSA discussed in Part 3 could explore this further.

In the same piece of research, McCartan (2016) interviewed stakeholders and discerned that professionals felt that CoSA had a positive impact upon Core Member reintegration and risk management. Professionals viewed the volunteers as a second set of eyes, often considering the volunteers as substitutes for themselves. The professionals felt that Core Members are more likely to open up to the volunteers and potentially give away information relating to their risk which they would otherwise refrain from discussing with professionals involved in their lives. Although the professionals were generally happy with the support provided by the volunteers, concerns were also raised about volunteers taking on too much responsibility on the accountability aspect of the CoSA. Some professionals believed that volunteers should concentrate on the supportive aspect of the CoSA, whilst allowing the professionals to lead on the accountability aspect. This was due to concerns that volunteers may be under qualified to hold the Core Member accountable, something which should remain with the professionals. Some professionals were also concerned that Core Members would be able to manipulate volunteers due to their lack of experience and training in the area of sexual offending, although volunteers themselves felt well equipped to cope with Core Members on the basis of the training they had received.

Volunteering is usually thought of positively. Raise the topic of voluntary work with a friend or family member and their immediate thoughts may turn to helping members of the public, assisting in community environmental schemes or charity work with animals. However, the stigma surrounding individuals with convictions of sexual offences may mean that volunteers who support Core Members may also be subject to stigma by way of association. One way in which volunteers of CoSA can defend against such stigma is through the argument that they are not only supporting individuals convicted of sexual offences but also holding them accountable for their offences. It could be argued that the accountability aspect is more necessary for community members than it is helpful for Core Members. It may be that the accountability aspect is used to allow volunteers to feel they are reducing risk of recidivism as well as offering support.

Research by Höing et al. (2015) has shown how some Core Members have dropped out of their CoSA through feeling accused and condemned by their volunteers. The same research also evidenced how Core Members dropped out when faced with volunteers who approached CoSA discussions with a confrontational style. Whilst research by Fox (2015) has shown that unsuccessful CoSA are those which focussed upon accountability. It could be argued that the Core Member does not need reminding of their accountability within the CoSA. If CoSA are to be a strength based approach, the needs of the Core Member must come first. At present volunteers in CoSA that focus discussions around accountability rather than support are at best unnecessary and at worst damaging (Fox,

2015). Additionally, it would be beneficial to consider whether the accountability element encourages volunteer applications from individuals who naturally present a confrontational style and would therefore be deemed unsuitable.

Conclusion

The topics presented in this chapter can be used to evaluate the effectiveness of CoSA, both in terms of risk reduction in the community and the wellbeing of Core Members. It has been argued that there is not enough evidence to suggest that CoSA alone has the ability to reduce Core Members' recidivism risk. However, the limited research that has been carried out into the effect of CoSA on Core Members' emotional wellbeing suggests that Core Members do benefit from the support offered within CoSA. There is evidence to suggest that CoSA promotes positive psychosocial outcomes and improvements in certain psychosocial factors such as social support, which have been evidenced to promote desistance (Farmer, Beech, & Ward, 2012). If the CoSA construct is capable of promoting positive change in Core Members' emotional wellbeing, reduced recidivism may occur as a by-product.

Unfortunately, not all CoSA are successful. Research into factors contributing toward premature and successful CoSA endings is needed to help improve knowledge and understanding. An in-depth analysis and consideration of both cohorts could be used to identify areas for service delivery improvements. Further research could also consider the challenges involved in CoSA and what can be done to successfully overcome such challenges. Finally, it has been suggested that an exploration into the experiences and perceptions of volunteers and coordinators could be used to improve CoSA practices whilst providing a complete picture of Circles UK. CoSA are not a treatment programme and cannot be used in place of such. However, if CoSA has the ability to contribute to a reduction in recidivism through the support of volunteers from the general public, the CoSA construct would prove to be invaluable.

References

Andrews, D. A., & Bonta, J. (2010). *The psychology of criminal conduct*. London: Routledge.

Bailey, D. J., & Sample, L. L. (2017). An examination of a cycle of coping with strain among registered citizens' families. *Criminal Justice Studies, 30*(2), 158–180. https://doi.org/10.1080/147eenn8601X.2017.1299286

Bates, A., & Wager, N. (2016, September). *Analysis of the dynamic risk review and adverse outcomes for Circles Core Members*. Paper presented at the European Criminology Conference at Munster University, Germany.

Bates, A., Williams, D., Wilson, C., & Wilson, R. J. (2013). Circles South East: The first 10 years 2002–2012. *International Journal of Offender Therapy and Comparative Criminology, 58*(7), 861–885. https://doi.org/10.1177/0306624X13485362

Baumeister, R. F., Campbell, J. D., Krueger, J. I., & Vohs, K. D. (2003). Does high self-esteem cause better performance, interpersonal success, happiness, or healthier lifestyles? *Psychological Science in the Public Interest, 4*(1), 1–44. https://doi.org/10.1111/1529-1006.01431

Beech, A. R., Fisher, D. D., & Thornton, D. (2003). Risk assessment of sex offenders. *Professional Psychology: Research and Practice, 34*(4), 339–352.

Beyko, M. J., & Wong, S. C. (2005). Predictors of treatment attrition as indicators for program improvement not offender shortcomings: A study of sex offender treatment attrition. *Sexual Abuse: A Journal of Research and Treatment, 17*(4), 375–389. https://doi.org/10.1177/107906320501700403

Blagden, N. J., Winder, B., Thorne, K., & Gregson, M. (2011). 'No-one in the world would ever wanna speak to me again': An interpretative phenomenological analysis into convicted sexual offenders' accounts and experiences of maintaining and leaving denial. *Psychology, Crime & Law, 17*(7), 563–585. https://doi.org/10.1080/10683160903397532

Clarke, M., Brown, S., & Völlm, B. (2015). Circles of support and accountability for sex offenders: A systematic review of outcomes. *Sexual Abuse: A Journal of Research and Treatment*, 1–33. https://doi.org/10.1177/1079063215603691

de Vries Robbé, M., Mann, R. E., Maruna, S., & Thornton, D. (2015). An exploration of protective factors supporting desistance from sexual offending. *Sexual Abuse, 27*(1), 16–33. https://doi.org/10.1177/1079063214547582

Elliott, I. A., Beech, A. R., Mandeville-Norden, R., & Hayes, E. (2009). Psychological profiles of internet sexual offenders. *Sexual Abuse, 21*(1), 76–92. https://doi.org/10.1177/1079063208326929

Farmer, M., Beech, A. R., & Ward, T. (2012). Assessing desistance in child sexual abusers: A qualitative study. *Journal of Interpersonal Violence, 27*(5), 930–950. https://doi.org/10.1177/0886260511423255

Fox, K. J. (2015). Contextualizing the policy and pragmatics of reintegrating sex offenders. *Sexual Abuse: A Journal of Research and Treatment, 29*(1), 28–50. https://doi.org/10.1177/1079063215574711

Fox, K. J. (2016). Civic commitment: Promoting desistance through community integration. *Punishment & Society, 18*(1), 68–94. https://doi.org/10.1177/1462474515623102

Hanson, R. K., Gordon, A., Harris, A. J., Marques, J. K., Murphy, W., Quinsey, V. L., et al. (2002). First report of the collaborative outcome data project on the effectiveness of psychological treatment for sex offenders. *Sexual Abuse: A Journal of Research and Treatment, 14*(2), 169–194. https://doi.org/10.1177/107906320201400207

Hanson, R. K., & Hanson, R. K. (2007). *Assessing the risk of sexual offenders on community supervision: The Dynamic Supervision Project* 5(6). Ottawa, ON: Public Safety Canada.

Hanson, R. K., Harris, A. J. R., Helmus, L., & Thornton, D. (2014). High-risk sex offenders may not be high risk forever. *Journal of Interpersonal Violence, 29*(15), 2792–2813. https://doi.org/10.1177/0886260514526062

Harper, C. A., & Hogue, T. E. (2015). The emotional representation of sexual crime in the national British press. *Journal of Language and Social Psychology, 34*(1), 3–24. https://doi.org/10.1177/0261927X14544474

Höing, M., Bogaerts, S., & Vogelvang, B. (2016). Helping sex offenders to desist offending: The gains and drains for CoSA volunteers—A review of the literature. *Sexual Abuse, 28*(5), 364–402. https://doi.org/10.1177/1079063214535816

Höing, M., Vogelvang, B., & Bogaerts, S. (2015). "I am a different man now"—Sex offenders in circles of support and accountability a prospective study. *International Journal of Offender Therapy and Comparative Criminology, 61*(7), 751–772. https://doi.org/10.1177/0306624X15612431

Larochelle, S., Diguer, L., Laverdière, O., & Greenman, P. S. (2011). Predictors of psychological treatment noncompletion among sexual offenders. *Clinical Psychology Review, 31*(4), 554–562.

Malinen, S., Willis, G. M., & Johnston, L. (2014). Might informative media reporting of sexual offending influence community members' attitudes towards sex offenders? *Psychology, Crime & Law, 20*(6), 535–552. https://doi.org/10.1080/1068316X.2013.793770

Mann, R. E., Hanson, R. K., & Thornton, D. (2010). Assessing risk for sexual recidivism: Some proposals on the nature of psychologically meaningful risk factors. *Sexual Abuse, 22*(2), 191–217.

Maslow, A. H. (1943). A theory of human motivation. *Psychological Review, 50*(4), 370–396. https://doi.org/10.1037/h0054346

McAnena, C., Craissati, J., & Southgate, K. (2016). Exploring the role of locus of control in sex offender treatment. *Journal of Sexual Aggression, 22*(1), 95–106. https://doi.org/10.1080/13552600.2015.1023374

McCartan, K. (2016). *Circles of support and accountability: Cabinet office—Social Action Fund evaluation.* Project report. University of the West of England, Bristol, UK. Retrieved from http://eprints.uwe.ac.uk/28279

Mingus, W., & Burchfield, K. B. (2012). From prison to integration: Applying modified labeling theory to sex offenders. *Criminal Justice Studies, 25*(1), 97–109. https://doi.org/10.1080/1478601X.2012.657906

Moore, G. F., Audrey, S., Barker, M., Bond, L., Bonell, C., Hardeman, W., et al. (2015). Process evaluation of complex interventions: Medical Research Council guidance. *BMJ, 350*. https://doi.org/10.1136/bmj.h1258

Pearlin, L., & Schooler, C. (1978). The structure of coping. *Journal of Health and Social Behavior, 19*(1), 2–21.

Purvis, M., Ward, T., & Willis, G. (2011). The good lives model in practice: Offence pathways and case management. *European Journal of Probation, 3*(2), 4–28. https://doi.org/10.1177/206622031100300202

Rotter, J. B. (1966). Generalized expectancies for internal versus external control of reinforcement. *Psychological Monographs: General and Applied, 80*(1), 1–28. https://doi.org/10.1037/h0092976

Ryan, R. M., & Deci, E. L. (2001). On happiness and human potential: A review of research on hedonic and eudaimonic well-being. *Annual Review of Psychology, 52*(1), 141–166. https://doi.org/10.1146/annurev.psych.52.1.141

Schmitt, M. T., Branscombe, N. R., Postmes, T., & Garcia, A. (2014). The consequences of perceived discrimination for psychological well-being: A meta-analytic review. *Psychological Bulletin, 140*(4), 921–948. https://doi.org/10.1037/a0035754

Schultz, C. (2014). The stigmatization of individuals convicted of sex offenses: Labeling theory and the sex offense registry. *Themis: Research Journal of Justice Studies and Forensic Science, 2*(1), 1–18.

Sullivan, S. A., Thompson, A., Kounali, D., Lewis, G., & Zammit, S. (2017). The longitudinal association between external locus of control, social cognition and adolescent psychopathology. *Social Psychiatry and Psychiatric Epidemiology, 52*(643), 1–13. https://doi.org/10.1007/s00127-017-1359-z

Swinburne Romine, R. E., Miner, M. H., Poulin, D., Dwyer, S. M., & Berg, D. (2012). Predicting reoffense for community-based sexual offenders: An analysis of 30 years of data. *Sexual Abuse, 24*(5), 501–514. https://doi.org/10.1177/1079063212446514

Tennant, R., Hiller, L., Fishwick, R., Platt, S., Joseph, S., Weich, S., et al. (2007). The Warwick-Edinburgh mental well-being scale (WEMWBS): Development and UK validation. *Health and Quality of life Outcomes, 5*(1), 1–13. https://doi.org/10.1186/1477-7525-5-63

Thornton, D. (2002). Constructing and testing a framework for dynamic risk assessement. *Sexual Abuse: A Journal of Research and Treatment, 14*(2), 139–153. https://doi.org/10.1177/107906320201400205

Watson, R., Thomas, S., & Daffern, M. (2015). The impact of interpersonal style on ruptures and repairs in the therapeutic alliance between offenders and therapists in sex offender treatment. *Sexual Abuse: A Journal of Research and Treatment*, 1–20. https://doi.org/10.1177/1079063215617514

Wilson, R. J., McWhinnie, A. J., & Wilson, C. (2008). Circles of support and accountability: An international partnership in reducing sexual offender recidivism. *Prison Service Journal, 138*(178), 26–36.

6

The Role of the Media in Shaping Responses to Sexual Offending

Craig A. Harper

A number of authors have commented on the role of the media in shaping and reinforcing attitudes and perceptions of people convicted of sexual offences (Harper & Hogue, 2017; King & Roberts, 2017; Soothill & Walby, 1991). In these works, the general idea is that the media produces a stereotypical image of who such perpetrators might be, and then continue to cover selective and sensationalised stories involving individuals who match this stereotype. Until recently, the psychological processes underpinning these practices were not well understood, or researched in any meaningful way. This chapter explores some emerging evidence about the psychological mechanisms that are invoked by such media practices, and unpacks some contemporary debates about who 'sexual offenders' (in this chapter, these individuals are referred to as 'individuals who have committed sexual offences') are, how they are represented, and what effect this has on social discussions about the prevention of sexual crime. In doing so, these ideas are related specifically to Circles of Support and Accountability projects ('Circles'/CoSA) throughout the chapter.

C. A. Harper (✉)
Nottingham Trent University, Nottingham, UK

H. Elliott et al. (eds.), *Sexual Crime and Circles of Support and Accountability*, Sexual Crime, https://doi.org/10.1007/978-3-319-74823-8_6

Psychological Processes in Media Reporting of Sexual Offending

As stated above, the media—particularly national news outlets—have been commonly cited as drivers of social attitudes towards individuals who have committed sexual offences. In the most recent analyses of these effects, it has been reported that British tabloid newspaper readers (e.g., those who read The Sun, The Daily Mirror, or The Daily Mail) expressed more negative views than broadsheet newspaper readers (e.g., those who read The Times, The Guardian, or The Daily Telegraph). Those who read a combination of these two newspaper types scored somewhere between the two 'exclusive' readership groups (Harper & Hogue, 2017). Importantly, these differences were present after controlling for well-known predictors of attitudes towards individuals who have committed sexual offences, such as participants' educational attainment. Thus, these findings indicate that there may be something inherent in the content of the sexual crime coverage in these publications that contributes to differences in attitudes. In this section, some of the psychological mechanisms that are at play when media outlets talk about sexual offending are unpacked. In particular, ideas related to non-conscious information processing will be explored, specifically in relation to how media outlets use heuristics to communicate about sexual crime.

Dual-Process Cognition: A Brief Introduction

Generally speaking, dual-process models of cognition assume that people use two mental 'systems' for processing information. One of these systems is automatic and non-conscious in nature, enabling people to form rapid judgements with little cognitive effort. The second system is more elaborative, and involves people using conscious reasoning, and the evaluation of available information, before making a decision (for a popular review of this research, see Kahneman, 2011).

Sigmund Freud (1923) first introduced a distinction between conscious and non-conscious cognitive processes to the psychological literature, suggesting that human information processing (which he referred to as psychic activity) occurred first at a non-conscious level (the 'primary process'; System 1), and later at the conscious level of awareness (the 'secondary process'; System 2). Building on Freud's conceptualisation of the primary and secondary process, numerous scholars have sought to introduce more cognitively-grounded dual-process models of information processing into the psychological literature. Examples of these models include Cognitive-Experiential Self-Theory (Epstein, 1994, 2003), the Elaboration Likelihood Model (Petty & Cacioppo, 1986), the Heuristic-Systematic Model (Chaiken, 1980), and System 1/System 2 Theory (Kahneman, 2011).

Each of these dual-process models begin with the assumption that we make decisions using two distinct mental systems. First, we have a quick, non-conscious system, which uses previous experience to formulate a range of heuristics in long-term memory. Heuristics are mental shortcuts that facilitate rapid decision-making when a stimulus is presented. By using heuristics, we can non-consciously evaluate the stimulus within the context of prior experience, and act accordingly with minimal cognitive effort being used. As such, these heuristics act as a cognitive framework around which we base our understanding, information processing, and decision-making in the real world. The most common heuristics include *availability*, *representativeness*, and *affect*. These three heuristics have been identified as having an important role to play in understanding people's responses to individuals who have committed sexual offences (Harris & Socia, 2016), and as such will be considered in more detail here.

The Availability Heuristic in Sexual Crime Coverage

The availability heuristic is a mental process whereby familiar or more common stimuli are processed more quickly than unfamiliar or less common stimuli. Tversky and Kahneman (1974) suggested that the ease at which a person can recall examples of particular categories determines how prevalent or important those categories are perceived as being. For example, people have been found to rate themselves as less assertive when asked to recall twelve occasions in which they had demonstrated this characteristic than participants who recall only six (Schwarz et al., 1991).

This finding is counter-intuitive, as recalling more examples should surely lead to increased perceptions of assertiveness. Schwarz et al. concluded that ratings of assertiveness were not driven by the *number* of cases recall, but rather by *how easily* the examples came to mind. The first six examples came to mind easily for all participants, but the trouble in naming six additional examples experienced by those having to recall twelve cases led them to doubt their level of assertiveness.

Media agenda-setting is one applied area that operates using the principle of availability. McCombs and Shaw (1972) reported a strong correlation between issues that their participants believed were politically important, and the rate at which these issues were reported in the news. Public perceptions of the nature and importance of a topic can be manipulated by "availability entrepreneurs" (Kuran & Sunstein, 1999, p. 687). These are stakeholders (who are typically news organisations or pressure groups) with a vested interest in a given topic, and an ability to change the direction of social discourse. In their *availability cascade* model, Kuran and Sunstein argued that availability entrepreneurs set the tone for particular topics, and increase media coverage of them. This increased coverage then amplifies societal views, causing the cascade to become a self-fulfilling prophecy. As such, the extent to which an issue is discussed at a societal level appears to have a link to how prevalent or important society views it as.

Perhaps the most high-profile case of availability cascades in operation in the area of sexual crime comes in the form of community notification laws. In the American context, the 1994 sexual murder of seven-year-old Megan Kanka by Jesse Timmendequas acted as a springboard for such policies to be introduced. Timmendequas was a neighbour of the Kanka family, and had a string of previous sexual convictions, including multiple sexual assaults against young girls. Kanka's parents, Richard and Maureen, started to campaign for community notification to be made a legal requirement in relation to those with previous convictions of this kind, arguing that their daughter would have still been alive had they known about Timmendequas' past. After first successfully lobbying local legislators in relation to sex offender registration and public disclosure of information, President Bill Clinton enacted federal legislation as part of the Jacob Wetterling Crimes

Against Children and Sexually Violent Offender Registration Act of 1994. Since then, police departments have been legally bound to require all individuals who have committed sexual offences to sign registries, and subsequently to make information about these individuals available to local communities. Exactly how this information is made available varies between states, but common practices include social media updates, public websites, local community leaflets, and smartphone applications.

The 2000 abduction and murder of Sarah Payne by Roy Whiting who, like Timmendequas, had convictions for sexual offences against children, led to a high-profile media campaign to introduce a "Megan's Law" style system in the UK. Alongside the *News of the World* newspaper (now defunct following the 2011–2012 press hacking scandal), the Payne family launched a national campaign in an attempt to force law enforcement officials to release information about where individuals who have committed sexual offences live. The pretence of this initiative, as in the campaign led by the Kanka family six years earlier, was that such a scheme would enable parents to protect their children from people they called 'sexual predators'. Repeated news coverage of the campaign for "Sarah's Law" led to widespread public support for community notification, with 82% of the British public supporting the introduction of the scheme in polling conducted in August 2000 (Ipsos Mori, 2000). Following ten years of debate, the Child Sex Offender Disclosure Scheme was piloted and subsequently enacted nationally, allowing concerned members of the public to apply to the police for information about the offending histories of individuals that they suspect of being a danger to local children. The police then have the option of disclosing any offence-related information about the suspected individual to a person best placed to protect local children (Home Office, 2010).

It is not only in high-profile political campaigning that the availability heuristic can be observed in social coverage of sexual crime. There was an approximately 300% increase in the coverage of convicted cases of sexual crime in British newspapers in the twelve months following the re-emergence of high-profile allegations of sexual offending being made against the deceased entertainer Jimmy Savile (Harper & Hogue, 2017). This was in spite of criteria being in place to exclude stories specifically about Jimmy Savile, and the numerous police operations stemming from this case, within this study. The presence of the Savile scandal in such a dataset that sought to specifically exclude it indicates the pervasive impact that individual high-profile cases can have on broader discussions about sexual crime. Further, the increase in sexual crime coverage occurred while coverage of non-sexual crimes remained comparatively stable. This led Harper and Hogue to conclude that the high-profile nature of the Jimmy Savile scandal led to sexual crime being seen as more newsworthy, providing evidence of availability processes being in operation at the level of news coverage.

The Representativeness Heuristic in Sexual Crime Coverage

The representativeness heuristic is a mental process whereby stimuli are intuitively categorised based on their closeness to stereotypes. When provided with a description of a quiet, conscientious, and solitary man, for example, people are more inclined to suggest that this man was, for example, a librarian rather than an airline pilot or salesperson (Tversky & Kahneman, 1974). This is in spite of there being far fewer librarians than members of the other occupational groups. Similarly, people are more likely to suggest that a mock student with a meticulous and orderly personality profile is an engineering student than a liberal arts student (Kahneman & Tversky, 1973). These outcomes were reported to be reflective of mental stereotypes that we all hold, whether consciously or unconsciously, about the types of people who are likely to engage in different types of careers.

The representativeness heuristic is not limited to judgements about occupations or education. Medical professionals make use of the heuristic in order to make diagnoses on the basis of the symptoms present within their patients (Groopman, 2008). This allows patients to visit their GPs and quickly receive effective medication for minor acute ailments. However, there are many dangers of the representativeness in this context, with the potential for incorrect diagnoses being made based upon the characteristics of patients rather than physical symptoms (Klein, 2005). These findings demonstrate the pervasiveness of heuristic-based decision-making in a range of contexts.

Within the context of sexual crime, "when asked about 'sex offenders' many are inclined to envision the media-proliferated stereotypical image of a violent, predatory male p[a]edophile" (King & Roberts, 2017, p. 72). The notion that particular stereotypical images come to mind automatically is in keeping with the representativeness heuristic. This claim has empirical support from a number of recent experimental studies. Harris and Socia (2016), for instance, found that people assessed punitive policy proposals more positively when framed as targeting 'sex offenders' than 'people who have committed crimes of a sexual nature'.

Although several studies have used media coverage of sexual crime to suggest the presence of stereotypes about this group of offenders (e.g., Sanghara & Wilson, 2006), whether such stereotypes actually exist in practice (and whether they have tangible effects on judgements and behaviour) is an unanswered question. Beginning to address this knowledge gap, Harper and Bartels (2016) examined the role of implicit theories (ITs; Dweck, Chui, & Hong, 1995) about individuals who have committed sexual offences in the processing of information about different perpetrator profiles. They found that those who expressed an entity-based IT (advocating the view that sexual offending is an innate and unchangeable aspect of a perpetrator's personality), viewed an adult male child abuser's offending behaviour as more indicative of his moral character, and more deserving of punishment than the actions of an adult female's or a juvenile's offending behaviour. In contrast, these judgements were broadly stable across the three perpetrator profiles among those participants expressing an incremental IT (where sexual offending is viewed as a changeable characteristic of an individual's personality).

In a separate analysis, holding an entity-based IT about individuals who have committed sexual offences strengthened the relationship between generalised attitudes towards this group and sentencing preferences for the adult male perpetrator (Harper & Bartels, 2017). This finding indicated that the presentation of a representative case example re-affirmed an implicitly-held stereotype about who 'sexual offenders' (as was the term used in the study) are among those with an entity IT, which in turn enhanced the relationship between generalised attitudes and sentencing judgements among these participants. These data converge to suggest that judgements about 'sexual offenders' (as a homogenous label) are primarily guided by the content and emotionality of some stereotypical (or *representative*) image of who these individuals actually are.

The Affect Heuristic in Sexual Crime Coverage

The affect heuristic is a mental process whereby decisions are made on the basis of automatic positive or negative feelings about a given object or issue (Slovic & Peters, 2006). On the stock market, for example, we typically make investments on the basis of how much we like or dislike particular brands, rather than their relative qualities (Kahneman, 2011; Zajonc, 1980). We also take this affect-based approach when making decisions about social and political phenomena. In perhaps one of the clearest examples of the affect heuristic, Finucane, Alhakami, Slovic, and Johnson (2000) used vignettes to manipulate the levels of risks or benefits associated with various energy technologies. They found that participants presented with 'high risk' information reported fewer benefits associated with these technologies, and those presented with 'high benefit' information reported fewer risks. This was in spite of only risk-based or benefit-based information being presented. In conclusion, Finucane et al. suggested that judgements of risk and benefit are implicitly linked, and that affect may be a driving force in social and political decision-making.

Alongside their findings that attitudes towards those convicted of sexual offences varies depending on the newspaper read, Harper and Hogue (2017) also examined data in relation to the specific differences between British national tabloids and broadsheets in the ways in which they reported on sexual crimes. Specifically, they used a piece of computer software called Linguistic Inquiry and Word Count (LIWC; Pennebaker, Chung, Ireland, Gonzales, & Booth, 2007) to examine articles in relation to their emotional content. In spite of the readership-based differences in attitudes towards individuals who have committed sexual offences between tabloid and broadsheet readers, these two types of publication did not differ on any of the emotional indices that were examined: negative emotionality, positive emotionality, anger, and anxiety. However, there were substantial differences in the descriptors used about individuals who have committed sexual offences in the headlines of articles. While tabloids used overtly hostile and disparaging headline descriptions of these individuals (e.g., "beast", "fiend", and "monster"), broadsheets were more measured in their labelling, using more neutral terms such as "man", "brother", or citing the occupations of those convicted of the crimes being reported.

With these findings in mind, it may be that the dehumanisation of those with convictions for sexual offences plays a contributing role in the formation and expression of negative attitudes towards these individuals. Dehumanisation is a core aspect of moral disengagement theory (Bandura, Barbaranelli, Caprara, & Pastorelli, 1996), which argues that people are able to sanction immoral behaviour by using a range of psychological and linguistic mechanisms. That is, decision-making in relation to politically-sensitive topics are grounded in affect-based cognitive processes—not in accordance to what *ought* to be right (a rational mode of decision-making), but by what *feels* to be right (an intuitive mode of decision-making).

Although traditionally used to explain how people make politically-contentious decisions (e.g., support for military action), the mechanisms of moral disengagement may have some utility in understanding punitive responses to legal transgressions. Drake and Henley (2014) discussed the creation of a so-called "false dichotomy" (p. 141) between the rights of 'victims' and 'offenders' in social and political discourses about crime. They observed that the human rights of offenders are consistently placed in competition with those of their victims in political discourse. In this sense, the linguistically manufactured competitive distinction between victims and offenders serves only to promote ever-increasingly punitive responses to crime, and fulfils a populist need to increase the severity of criminal sanctions.

Specifically in relation to judgements of individuals who have committed sexual offences, dehumanisation (as measured by attributing non-human descriptors to the label 'sex offenders', has been associated with support for the social exclusion of those with sexual convictions, as well as for harsh punishments (including direct physical violence; Viki, Fullerton, Raggett, Tait, & Wiltshire, 2012). Similarly, child molesters were significantly more dehumanised than other offender groups, with dehumanisation being positively associated with preferences for severe prison sentences, and negatively associated with views about the suitability of rehabilitative alternatives to custody (Bastian, Denson, & Haslam, 2013).

Bringing all of these findings together, it appears that viscerally-driven, intuitive emotional responses to the 'sex offender' label may be responsible for particularly negative responses towards these groups of individuals. Using this kind of framework also explains Harris and Socia's (2016) work on the effects of the 'sex offender' label. That is, views about "sex offenders" are contaminated with the emotion attached to this label, which may be driven by dehumanised attributions that are promoted in mainstream media outlets. In contrast, more descriptive and person-oriented language (e.g., "people who have committed crimes of a sexual nature" or "people with a sexual interest in children") do not illicit the same stereotypes or emotional responses, leading to more measured responses through rationally-based decision-making.

Public Views About CoSA and the Social Reintegration of People with Sexual Convictions

There is a public desire for strict punishments and effective treatments for individuals convicted of sexual crime (West, 2000), although recent press attention has been focused on the former of these. For example, in 2010 the UK Supreme Court ruled that it was a human right of individuals who have committed sexual offences to have the opportunity to appeal that they are no longer a risk to the public, and for their details to be removed from the Violent and Sexual Offenders Register (ViSOR). This ruling was met with widespread political and public condemnation, with the coalition government at the time claiming that it would make the minimum amount of changes to current registration procedures in order to meet the new requirements (BBC News, 2011).

Students have been found to express a preference for a combination of imprisonment and therapy as a sentence for individuals who have committed sexual offences (Koulianou, 1985). Similarly, Brown (1999) reported findings from a public survey in Wales that suggested high support for prison-based treatment programmes. However, when examining community-based treatment procedures, around 45% of Brown's sample thought that treatment for these individuals should take place *only* within a prison setting. Further, 80% of respondents to this study believed that only using community-based treatment procedures as a sentence for sexual offending would be a lenient approach to take, with around 90% rejecting this as a sentencing option entirely. These data all converge around a similar view—there is a public wish to see individuals who have committed sexual offences punished *and* rehabilitated within a prison setting.

This apparent support for rehabilitative schemes is a good thing, and highlights a public awareness of the utility of social reintegration. However, support for such procedures appears to drop when people are asked about these schemes taking place within their own communities (Brown, 1999). This 'Not-In-My-Backyard' style of thinking (NIMBYism) is not unique to the area of the treatment of individuals who have committed sexual offences. However, this lack of distinctiveness aside, NIMBYism breeds an 'Us vs. Them' approach, which has tangible effects on successful desistance processes (e.g., Göbbels, Ward, & Willis, 2012).

Looking at NIMBYism in more detail, those who hold the sexual crime prototypes of 'rapists' or 'paedophiles' (the most common labels used to describe individuals who have committed sexual offences within UK press reports; Harper & Hogue, 2015) express the highest levels of objection to the local rehousing of these individuals (Cook & Hogue, 2013). This response can be explained to some degree through the emotionally-charged activation of sexual crime prototypes that are promulgated by media outlets, with local people asking 'why should we accept people like *X* into our community?'. In this case, we can see how the emotional processing of high-profile cases contributes to blanket judgement. This explanation thus demonstrates the roles of both the affect and availability heuristics in decision-making about the social reintegration and rehabilitation of individuals who have committed sexual offences.

One potential shortcoming of some of the research noted above is that the focus has been on looking at support for 'treatment facilities' within local communities. In the present context, though, socially-oriented rehabilitation procedures are more likely to take the form of CoSA once people with sexual convictions have been released from custody.

Circles work by matching trained community volunteers to "Core Members", with volunteers offering social and practical support to the Core Member as they transition back into the community. Broadly, there appears to be widespread support for CoSA as a way of rehabilitating individuals who have committed sexual offences (e.g., McAvoy, 2012; Wilson, Picheca, & Prinzo, 2007). That is, around 70% of respondents in a number of public surveys saw value in these schemes, with only small numbers being suspicious about its aims or efficacy.

In spite of this early work suggesting social support for the CoSA model of reintegration, findings reported by Richards and McCartan (2017) may suggest that the framing of information about CoSA impacts upon such views. They examined social media comments made in response to online posts about the launch of CoSA in Australia. While they found that the comments were overwhelmingly hostile towards the idea of CoSA, it must be acknowledged that the framing of the initial posts were negatively-valenced (e.g., "Controversial paedophile support program to launch in South Australia in a national first", and "Stop the COSA Trial in South Australia Immediately"). With this in mind, it appears that focusing on the core messages about CoSA—particularly in relation to producing positively-framed messages about these procedures—is important, "given the strong negative reaction to the image of "supporting" child sex offenders" (Richards & McCartan, 2017, p. 13).

In spite of generally broad support for CoSA, there is a reluctance to actively and personally engage in CoSA procedures by many individuals. In one survey, over half of respondents (55%) said that they would support a friend who wanted to volunteer with CoSA, though only 12% would consider doing so themselves (Höing, Petrina, Duke, Völlm, & Vogelvang, 2016). It could be argued that this practice reflects a form of 'social NIMBYism'. As such, trends of supporting but not facilitating the treatment and rehabilitation of individuals who have committed sexual offences in the community requires more research. The aim of this research should be to understand these behaviours and encourage voluntary participation in CoSA arrangements.

Applying the theoretical work described earlier in this chapter to the specific context of CoSA, the presence of intuitive styles of thinking in relation to social discussions about sexual crime poses specific challenges for running and maintaining effective Circles. For instance, the recruitment of volunteers to CoSA schemes is dependent on a willingness of members of the public to come forward to work constructively and collaboratively with people who have convictions for sexual offences. The widespread availability of the 'monstrous sex offender' stereotype may act as a potential barrier to such recruitment efforts. It may be the case that those who may otherwise consider assisting with charitable organisations are averse to facilitating the smooth reintegration of former offenders like Jesse Timmendequas or Roy Whiting.

This aversion could come about for several reasons. The first and most obvious reason may be rooted in potential volunteers' own psychological intuitions. Sexual offending evokes an automatic visceral reaction. As Bastian et al. (2013) describe, we tend to experience instinctual emotional responses such as fear, loathing, and disgust when we are confronted by the details of sexual crime. These may even be associated with innate moral impulses related to care for the vulnerable, and to sexual purity (Harper & Harris, 2017).

Such reactions psychologically contribute to avoidance-based behaviours. That is, humans have a tendency to move away from those things they fear (Elliot, 2006). This framework can help us to understand how and why the 'social NIMBY' response occurs. Generalised emotional responses, when coupled with high-profile exemplars around which to tangibly frame moral arguments, may contribute to a rejection of CoSA volunteering opportunities among those who may otherwise be perfect candidates for supporting people with sexual convictions back into the community.

With this in mind, it is important to consider the ways in which attitudes towards people with sexual convictions might be changed. From the review presented earlier in this chapter, targeting automatic emotional responses that are rooted in heuristic information processing may be the most effective way to improve social responses to these individuals.

As such, the remainder of this chapter considers how researchers have sought to improve social attitudes towards people who have committed sexual offences, and how CoSA may have an important role to play in these efforts.

Using the Media to Change Attitudes towards Individuals Who Have Committed Sexual Offences

Considering the above work, it is clear that improving societal attitudes towards (the rehabilitation and reintegration of) individuals who have committed sexual offences would be of huge benefit, at both the individual and social levels, and that CoSA initiatives have a major role to play in these processes.

The implicit aim of much of this research appears to have been to identify potential between-groups differences on the part of those providing their views, and to begin to formulate strategies for influencing these views. While the long-term effectiveness of attitude change efforts—particularly at the macro level—have not been extensively examined, there have been some successful laboratory and survey-based approaches that appear to have some potential utility in this regard.

Malinen, Willis, and Johnston (2014) directly examined the malleability of public attitudes towards individuals who have committed sexual offences via the media using manipulations of mock news stories. They found that people presented with an 'informative' mock news story (which presented structured information about an individual's risk assessments) expressed significantly more positive attitudes towards individuals who have committed sexual offences than participants who just provided their attitudes without reading a story. However, there was no difference in the attitudes between participants presented with the 'informative' story or a more 'typical' (emotionally-driven) alternative, indicating that merely being presented with any kind of news story about an individual who has committed a sexual offence led to a deterioration in attitudes when compared to those who were not primed with a story.

An interesting addition to Malinen et al.'s design was the inclusion of a measure of implicit attitudes, where participants were asked to link 'positive' and 'negative' words with a particular attitude target (in this case, 'sexual offenders') as fast as they can using a computer keyboard. This procedure represents a direct test of the affect heuristic as reported previously in this chapter. No significant differences in the speed of response were reported on this measure as a function of the type of mock news story that participants read. This indicated that the different news presentations did not influence the automatic evaluations about individuals who have committed sexual offences that were held by participants in their study. The authors concluded that, while there is potential to influence public attitudes towards this group through media presentations, repeated exposure to information targeted at emotional responses to sexual crime may be needed to achieve reliable and long-lasting attitude change.

While this work represents an important first step in identifying the role of the media in changing attitudes towards individuals who have committed sexual offences, it is unavoidable to ignore some of its limitations. The most important of these is that the focus was predominantly on *explicit* rather than *implicit* cognition. That is, by reading an 'informative' or 'emotional' piece about an individual who had committed a sexual offence, participants were being asked to consciously consider their views.

As highlighted earlier in this chapter, there is an emerging evidence base that attitudes towards individuals who have committed sexual offences, as well as views about their treatment and management, are rooted in non-conscious implicit cognition. With this in mind, it is important for researchers to build this premise in to their studies—and more importantly in to their experimental stimuli—in order to examine whether more indirect communication methods can contribute to attitude improvement.

One area where this approach has been used is in relation to views about people with paedophilic sexual interests. While not synonymous with 'sexual offenders', these individuals are typically associated with sexual offending behaviour through media presentations (Feelgood & Hoyer, 2008). In addition, analyses of newspaper headlines suggested that these individuals are heavily dehumanised within the press, with this being a potential driver of negative attitudes via the affect heuristic (Harper & Hogue, 2017). With this in mind, it is perhaps a constructive step to investigate whether the affect-based *re*humanisation of individuals who have committed sexual offences could lead to improvements in social attitudes.

Two studies have sought to examine rehumanisation in relation to paedophiles. In the first, participants presented with information about paedophiles from the perspective of somebody with a sexual interest in children expressed significant improvements in their explicit (self-reported) attitudes towards this group as compared to a control group, who were presented with a video about violence-free parenting (Jahnke, Philipp, & Hoyer, 2015). Moreover, this effect was still present in follow-up testing six weeks after the experimental manipulation, indicating a stable change in viewpoints over time as a result of this intervention.

Harper, Bartels, and Hogue (2016) went further by directly isolating the source of the message from the message itself. They used a video clip from the British Documentary *The Paedophile Next Door*, which told the story of 'Eddie' (a pseudonym)—a man living every day as a non-offending self-identifying paedophile. He spoke of the stigma he faces, the need for social support, and how policies could be put in place to prevent sexual offending before it occurs. This represented a humanising approach. A separate group were presented with a video clip of an expert speaking of the nature of paedophilia, and concluding with similar claims about the best ways to prevent sexual abuse. By adopting such an approach, this study was able to identify whether it was indeed the humanisation element of Jahnke et al.'s manipulation, rather than the content of the message, that led to significantly improved attitudes.

Both groups demonstrated significant reductions in negative attitudes towards paedophiles, though this effect was far greater in the humanising condition. Even more interestingly, the narrative-based humanisation of Eddie's clip led to more positive responding at the implicit level than did the expert-delivered information. This result highlights the potential utility of direct exposure to examples of potential offenders that run counter to media stereotypes when attempting to influence attitudes.

This idea supports theoretical arguments made by some criminologists, who have highlighted society's lack of a desistance narrative for individuals who have committed sexual offences (e.g., Farmer, McAlinden, & Maruna, 2015). That is, we typically do not hear from those who have been convicted for these types of offences—either about the precursors to their offending behaviour, or their journeys towards desistance. Again this has links to the heuristics discuss previously. If all that is available is a punitive and dehumanised 'monster' narrative, it is no surprise that lay members of the public jump to conclusions and make snap judgements based on this stereotype. By incorporating the voices of individuals who have committed sexual offences into mainstream discussions about sexual crime, we may be able to disrupt this tendency of heuristic decision-making and facilitate more rational discussions about the prevention of sexual crime.

The Way Forward: Incorporating Attitude Research into CoSA Practice

At the broadest level, it could be argued that being actively engaged in a functional Circle enables a Core Member to maintain a rehabilitation-reinforcing environment that is so important to the desistance process (Göbbels et al., 2012). This in turn contributes to the achievement of 'primary human goods'—broadly defined as intrinsic life goals that, if pursued and acquired, lead to the "actualization of potentialities that are distinctively human" (Ward & Gannon, 2006, p. 83). From a cursory examination of the GLM's primary human goods, it is clear that addressing the public's negative attitudes and reforming the ways in which individuals who have committed sexual offences are managed within the community after serving their criminal sentences should be considered as important areas for achieving re-entry and normalcy.

At the level of policymaking and support, lifelong registration procedures (and their associated restrictions) limit the opportunities for people with sexual convictions to achieve the goods of 'excellence in play', 'excellence in work', or 'excellence in agency'. This is because they are not free to exercise autonomy in relation to where they live, socialise, or work. Added to this is the perhaps heuristically-driven decision-making of landlords to not rent properties to these individuals (Clark, 2007), or employers to not offer them work opportunities (Brown, Spencer, & Deakin, 2007), which further compound the social difficulties faced by people with sexual convictions in relation to societal reintegration. Further, efforts to achieving close ties with other people (and thus the achievement of the primary goods of 'relatedness' and 'community') are hindered through the effects of the lifelong carrying of the 'sexual offender' label. These difficulties subsequently limit the extent to which goods such as 'inner peace' and 'pleasure' can be achieved. This risks feelings of hopelessness and self-stigma, which are associated with sexual recidivism (Levenson & Cotter, 2005).

The CoSA model is designed to intervene with and overcome these barriers, by providing social (e.g., friendship, access to activities) and practical (e.g., assistance with obtaining financial products and housing) support to Core Members in the immediate aftermath of their incarceration. Naturally, Circles are dependent on the availability, willingness, and commitment of volunteers to come forward and enact their role in a professional and effective way. These volunteers are drawn from the general community, and so there may be difficulties in recruiting such individuals in the face of widespread negativity towards this group of offenders. With this in mind, it may be possible to embed some of the humanisation strategies emerging from recent research into existing recruitment strategies (Harper et al., 2016; Jahnke et al., 2015). For instance, could potential Core Members act as the human face of the 'sex offender' label when discussing the need for volunteers? The findings of these early studies suggest that using real examples of people in need of support as they move away from sexual offending can have a powerful impact on broader attitudes. Further examples of how CoSA can promote its successes is through the wider dissemination of 'success stories'. That is, instead of promoting low reoffending figures, which require conscious elaboration of facts and statistics through 'System 2' cognition, CoSA might instead promote individual narrative examples of success more widely, this information is likely to be processed at a deeper (emotional) level, and contribute to longer-term improvements in social attitudes.

In short, if the research evidence around how to best influence attitudes towards individuals who have committed sexual offences can be incorporated into CoSA recruitment drives, there is a strong possibility that more volunteers could be brought in to CoSA schemes. This has subsequent effects for Core Members in terms of providing them with a supportive rehabilitative environment, and for the wider community in relation to keeping potential victims safe from harm.

Conclusions

This chapter has outlined the various ways in which the media influence public attitudes towards individuals who have committed sexual offences, and how these attitudes have subsequent effects on desistance-promoting schemes like CoSA. In short, it can be summarised under the following brief points:

1. Media outlets portray individuals who have committed sexual offences in such a way that encourages the public to base decisions on the rapid and heuristically-driven evaluations of selective case examples.
2. Public attitudes have an important role to play in the desistance processes of people with convictions for sexual offences, primarily through creating a rehabilitation-reinforcing environment within which they can move towards living a crime-free life.
3. There is broad public support for rehabilitative and preventative schemes like CoSA at the policy level, but a diffusion of responsibility at the individual level.
4. Academic research into attitudes towards individuals who have committed sexual offences and practice-based CoSA policies should be brought together to formulate more effective ways of bringing potential volunteers around Core Members.

References

Bandura, A., Barbaranelli, C., Caprara, G. V., & Pastorelli, C. (1996). Mechanisms of moral disengagement in the exercise of moral agency. *Journal of Personality and Social Psychology, 71*, 364–374. https://doi.org/10.1037/0022-3514.71.2.364

Bastian, B., Denson, T. F., & Haslam, N. (2013). The roles of dehumanization and moral outrage in retributive justice. *Plos One, 8*, e61842. https://doi.org/10.1371/journal.pone.0061842

BBC News. (2011). *Sex offender registration appeals to go ahead.* Retrieved April 28, 2017, from http://www.bbc.co.uk/news/uk-12476979

Brown, K., Spencer, J., & Deakin, J. (2007). The reintegration of sex offenders: Barriers and opportunities for employment. *The Howard Journal of Criminal Justice, 46*, 32–42. https://doi.org/10.1111/j.1468-2311.2007.00452.x

Brown, S. (1999). Public attitudes towards the treatment of sex offenders. *Legal and Criminological Psychology, 4*, 239–252. https://doi.org/10.1348/135532599167879

Chaiken, S. (1980). Heuristic versus systematic information processing and the use of source versus message cues in persuasion. *Journal of Personality and Social Psychology, 39*, 752–766. https://doi.org/10.1037/0022-3514.39.5.752

Clark, L. M. (2007). Landlord attitudes toward renting to released offenders. *Federal Probation, 71*, 20–30.

Cook, L., & Hogue, T. (2013, June). *Not-In-My-Backyard! A comparison of NIMBY responses to wind turbines and sex offender rehabilitation facilities.* Paper presented at the BPS Division of Forensic Psychology Annual Conference, Belfast, UK.

Drake, D. H., & Henley, A. J. (2014). 'Victims' versus 'offenders' in British political discourse: The construction of a false dichotomy. *The Howard Journal of Criminal Justice, 53*, 141–157. https://doi.org/10.1111/hojo.12057

Dweck, C. S., Chiu, C., & Hong, Y. (1995). Implicit theories and their role in judgments and reactions: A world from two perspectives. *Psychological Inquiry, 6*, 267–285. https://doi.org/10.1207/s15327965pli0604_1

Elliot, A. J. (2006). The hierarchical model of approach-avoidance motivation. *Motivation and Emotion, 30*, 111–116. https://doi.org/10.1007/s11031-006-9028-7

Epstein, S. (1994). An integration of the cognitive and psychodynamic unconscious. *American Psychologist, 49*, 709–724.

Epstein, S. (2003). Cognitive-experiential self-theory: An integrative theory of personality. In T. Millon & M. J. Lerner (Eds.), *Handbook of psychology: Personality and social psychology* (Vol. 5, pp. 93–118). Hoboken, NJ: John Wiley.

Farmer, M., McAlinden, A.-M., & Maruna, S. (2015). Understanding desistance from sexual offending: A thematic review of research findings. *Probation Journal, 62*, 320–335. https://doi.org/10.1177/0264550515600545

Feelgood, S., & Hoyer, J. (2008). Child molester or paedophile? Sociolegal versus psychopathological classification of sexual offenders against children. *Journal of Sexual Aggression, 14*, 33–43. https://doi.org/10.1080/13552600802133860

Finucane, M. L., Alhakami, A., Slovic, P., & Johnson, S. M. (2000). The affect heuristic in judgments of risks and benefits. *Journal of Behavioral Decision Making, 13*, 1–17. https://doi.org/10.1002/(SICI)1099-0771(200001/03)13:1<1::AID-BDM333>3.0.CO;2-S

Freud, S. (1923). *The ego and the id.* Vienna, Austria: W. W. Norton & Company.

Göbbels, S., Ward, T., & Willis, G. W. (2012). An integrative theory of desistance from sex offending. *Aggression and Violent Behavior, 17*, 453–462. https://doi.org/10.1016/j.avb.2012.06.003

Groopman, J. (2008). *How doctors think.* New York, NY: Houghton Mifflin Company.

Harper, C. A., & Bartels, R. M. (2016). Implicit theories and offender representativeness in judgments about sexual crime. *Sexual Abuse: A Journal of Research and Treatment.* Advanced online publication. https://doi.org/10.1177/1079063216658019

Harper, C. A., & Bartels, R. M. (2017). The influence of implicit theories and offender characteristics on judgements of sexual offenders: A moderated mediation analysis. *Journal of Sexual Aggression, 23*, 139–150. https://doi.org/10.1080/13552600.2016.1250963

Harper, C. A., Bartels, R. M., & Hogue, T. E. (2016). Reducing stigma and punitive attitudes toward pedophiles through narrative humanization. *Sexual Abuse: A Journal of Research and Treatment.* Advanced online publication. https://doi.org/10.1177/1079063216681561

Harper, C. A., & Harris, A. J. (2017). Applying moral foundations theory to understanding public views of sexual offending. *Journal of Sexual Aggression, 23*, 111–123. https://doi.org/10.1080/13552600.2016.1217086

Harper, C. A., & Hogue, T. E. (2015). The emotional representation of sexual crime in the national British press. *Journal of Language and Social Psychology, 34*, 3–24. https://doi.org/10.1177/0261927X14544474

Harper, C. A., & Hogue, T. E. (2017). Press coverage as a heuristic guide for social decision-making about sexual offenders. *Psychology, Crime & Law, 23*, 118–134. https://doi.org/10.1080/1068316X.2016.1227816

Harris, A. J., & Socia, K. M. (2016). What's in a name? Evaluating the effects of the "sex offender" label on public beliefs and opinions. *Sexual Abuse: A Journal of Research and Treatment, 28*, 660–678. https://doi.org/10.1177/1079063214564391

Höing, M., Petrina, R., Duke, L., Völlm, B., & Vogelvang, B. (2016). Community support for sex offender rehabilitation in Europe. *European Journal of Criminology, 13*, 491–516.

Home Office. (2010). *Child sex offender (CSO) disclosure scheme guidance document*. London: Author.

Ipsos, M. (2000). *Naming & shaming poll.* Retrieved from https://www.ipsos-mori.com/researchpublications/researcharchive/1619/Naming-amp-Shaming-Poll.aspx

Jahnke, S., Philipp, K., & Hoyer, J. (2015). Stigmatizing attitudes towards people with pedophilia and their malleability among psychotherapists in training. *Child Abuse & Neglect, 40*, 93–102. https://doi.org/10.1016/j.chiabu.2014.07.008

Kahneman, D. (2011). *Thinking, fast and slow*. London, UK: Penguin.

Kahneman, D., & Tversky, A. (1973). On the psychology of prediction. *Psychological Review, 80*, 237–251. https://doi.org/10.1037/h0034747

King, L. L., & Roberts, J. J. (2017). The complexity of public attitudes toward sex crimes. *Victims & Offenders, 12*, 71–89. https://doi.org/10.1080/15564886.2015.1005266

Klein, J. G. (2005). Five pitfalls in decisions about diagnosis and prescribing. *British Medical Journal, 330*, 781–783. https://doi.org/10.1136/bmj.330.7494.781

Koulianou, Y. (1985). *Attitudes towards rape: A cross-cultural approach*. Unpublished master's thesis. Cardiff: University of Wales.

Kuran, T., & Sunstein, C. R. (1999). Availability cascades and risk regulation. *Stanford Law Review, 51*, 683–768.

Levenson, J. S., & Cotter, L. P. (2005). The effect of Megan's Law on sex offender reintegration. *Journal of Contemporary Criminal Justice, 21*, 49–66. https://doi.org/10.1177/1043986204271676

Malinen, S., Willis, G. W., & Johnston, L. (2014). Might informative media reporting of sexual offending influence community members' attitudes towards sex offenders? *Psychology, Crime & Law, 20*, 535–552. https://doi.org/10.1080/1068316X.2013.793770

McAvoy, J. (2012). *Birds of a feather? Irish public attitudes towards sex crime and sex offender reintegration. Is there a publically perceived scale of sexual deviance?* Unpublished master's thesis, Dublin Institute of Technology, Dublin.

McCombs, M., & Shaw, D. (1972). The agenda-setting function of mass media. *Public Opinion Quarterly, 36*, 176–187. https://doi.org/10.1086/267990

Pennebaker, J. W., Chung, C. K., Ireland, M., Gonzales, A., & Booth R. J. (2007). *The development and psychometric properties of LIWC 2007* (Software manual). Austin, TX: LIWC.net.

Petty, R. E., & Cacioppo, J. T. (1986). The elaboration likelihood model of persuasion. In L. Berkowitz (Ed.), *Advances in experimental social psychology* (Vol. 19, pp. 123–205). New York, NY: Academic Press.

Richards, K., & McCartan, K. (2017). Public views about reintegrating child sex offenders via Circles of Support and Accountability (COSA): A qualitative analysis. *Deviant Behavior*. Advanced online publication. https://doi.org/10.1080/01639625.2017.1304800

Sanghara, K. K., & Wilson, J. C. (2006). Stereotypes and attitudes about child sexual abusers: A comparison of experienced and inexperienced professionals in sex offender treatment. *Legal and Criminological Psychology, 11*, 229–244. https://doi.org/10.1348/135532505X68818

Schwarz, N., Bless, H., Stack, F., Klumpp, G., Rittenauer-Schatka, H., & Simons, A. (1991). Ease of retrieval as information: Another look at the availability heuristic. *Journal of Personality and Social Psychology, 61*, 195–202. https://doi.org/10.1037/0022-3514.61.2.195

Slovic, P., & Peters, E. (2006). Risk perception and affect. *Current Directions in Psychological Science, 15*, 322–325. https://doi.org/10.1111/j.1467-8721.2006.00461.x

Soothill, K., & Walby, S. (1991). *Sex crime in the news*. London, UK: Routledge.

Tversky, A., & Kahneman, D. (1974). Judgment under uncertainty: Heuristics and biases. *Science, 185*, 1124–1131. https://doi.org/10.1126/science.185.4157.1124

Viki, G. T., Fullerton, I., Raggett, H., Tait, F., & Wiltshire, S. (2012). The role of dehumanization in attitudes toward the social exclusion and rehabilitation of sex offenders. *Journal of Applied Social Psychology, 42*, 2349–2367. https://doi.org/10.1111/j.1559-1816.2012.00944.x

Ward, T., & Gannon, T. A. (2006). Rehabilitation, etiology, and self-regulation: The comprehensive good loves model of treatment for sexual offenders. *Aggression and Violent Behavior, 11*, 77–94. https://doi.org/10.1016/j.avb.2005.06.001

West, D. J. (2000). The sex crime: Deterioration more apparent than real? *European Journal on Criminal Policy and Research, 8*, 399–422. https://doi.org/10.1023/A:1008713919597

Wilson, R., Picheca, J., & Prinzo, M. (2007). Evaluating the effectiveness of professionally-facilitated volunteerism in the community-based management of high-risk sexual offenders: Part One: Effects on participants and stakeholders. *The Howard Journal of Criminal Justice, 46*, 289–302. https://doi.org/10.1111/j.1468-2311.2007.00475.x

Zajonc, R. B. (1980). Feeling and thinking: Preferences need no inferences. *American Psychologist, 35*, 151–175. https://doi.org/10.1037/0003-066X.35.2.151

7

A Different Life: The Experiences of Core Members and Volunteers on the Safer Living Foundations Circles of Support and Accountability

Dave Potter

The following is a series of interviews I undertook in May 2017 with two Core Members and one volunteer from the Safer Living Foundation's (SLF) Circles of Support and Accountability (CoSA). The aim of this chapter was to explore and understand a Core Member's point of view and experience of a Circle to understand how best to move our Circles forwards, to keep and enhance best practice and to identify where we can make improvements. This chapter is about letting the voice of the service user (Core Members) speak out. In this respect, this chapter is similar to the chapter by Terry Philpot in Hanvey, Philpot, and Wilson's (2011) book on CoSA and could be considered an extension of their work.

The method I used was to record an interview with the Core Members, asking them to give a brief overview of their lives and offending behaviour

Dave Potter is coordinator for the Safer Living Foundation's Community Circles of Support and Accountability.

D. Potter (✉)
Safer Living Foundation, Visits Centre, HMP Whatton, Nottingham, UK

H. Elliott et al. (eds.), *Sexual Crime and Circles of Support and Accountability*,
Sexual Crime, https://doi.org/10.1007/978-3-319-74823-8_7

in order to gain an impression of how they came to offend, and then to ask about their Circles' experiences, both positive and negative.

I also interviewed one experienced volunteer and asked how she came to be interested in volunteering for such a position and again, the positives and negatives of her time on the Circle. I feel it is important that we listen to what our volunteers have to tell us, so that we can understand what works and what needs revisiting.

Within this chapter I also share my experiences as coordinator of the SLF Circles project.

All interviewees freely and enthusiastically gave of their time, and were open and honest about their Circle journey. The Core Members were especially keen to partake in this exercise and, as we have seen on many occasions from multiple Core Members, they were only too happy to be able to 'give something back' to the Circles which had given them so much support.

The following interviews have been edited for content; all identifying references have been removed and the names of all those interviewed have been altered.

Core Member Perspectives

Core member: Pete
Age at time of interview: 61
Offence history: Indecent assaults against females under 16 yrs old
Circle status: Successfully completed in August 2016
Circle duration: 17 months/52 sessions.

I grew up in a small village; there wasn't even a pub or a shop in the village. I had what seemed to me to be a pretty normal childhood at the time. I was in the Army cadet force for a couple of years from the age of 15 and then I joined the junior leader regiment, the Royal armoured core. However I was discharged after a year as unsuitable for further military training. I was a bit of a cocky sod because I could march and drill and shoot and do everything. Because of this, I was getting bullied by the others.

I started hitting the bottle a bit, drinking and I was only 15 years old. This is why I was discharged. I came home back to Mother and Dad where I was seduced by my oldest brother's wife, they were split up at the time, and I was 16 yrs old. I'd had sex before with one of the local village girls when I was about 13 yrs old. I didn't know what was going on that first time but this time I did and it lasted a few months and I was still drinking.

I got married at 20 yrs old but that only lasted a couple of years. I had bad anger problems when I was younger, I was arrested and charged with ABH against her when I was 21.

Just before going to court for sentencing, I went out drinking with a few friends and had a crash on my motorcycle on the way home. I had multiple arm and leg injuries. Even in hospital I was drinking, my parents bought me drink in. I'm not blaming my parents for how I turned out though, it's all down to me. They were out working all the time so I and my brothers got to run riot.

It was pretty harsh punishment if you were naughty from my Mum and Dad. We'd all get the belt or slipper if we stepped out of line.

In 1984, aged 30 yrs old, I started experimenting with amphetamine; and then, what can I say, I'd already been smoking cannabis for a few years, and then went onto the amphetamine and basically it was a downwards spiral from then with drink and drugs.

I've since been diagnosed with depression and when the doctor diagnosed me, it was like a light bulb going off! Looking back, the drink and the drugs, although they are depressants, at the time they made me feel good and I think that's why I took the drugs and alcohol. Take more drugs and beer to get up, then you go further down and so on. I got arrested a few times for possessing amphetamines.

I was having one night stands back then, having lots of sex. At that time I didn't respect women, I wouldn't beat them up, but as for sex, anything went. I saw them as sexual objects. This was around the time I indecently assaulted one of my girlfriend daughters. It came to light in 1989; I went to court in 1990, I went guilty and got 3 years It wasn't sexual intercourse, it was touching and feeling that I was getting my pleasure from and that's all that mattered to me at that time, I was selfish, not respecting women and I wanted my pleasure all the time. What I wanted and needed, that mattered and nothing else did. It was just a lack of respect for females and seeing them as sexual objects. In the last couple of years, since leaving prison I've been thinking a lot about why I did it, and that's the best answer I can find, the one that seems to fit.

In prison there was no therapy, no programmes, nothing and that's what pisses me off about the prison service back then. It was just *'welcome to prison, there's your cell'*. They'd lock the door and six months later or whatever they say *'off you go, there's your discharge grant and travel warrant, and we'll see you later!'* There was no rehabilitation, nothing!

When I got out, I was back on the drink and drugs, the downward spiral again. I was taking cannabis, cocaine, crack cocaine, cannabis, and ecstasy; around this time I was also selling drugs to people and I used to lose days at a time, I was that far out of it. I was working as a doorman on good money, dealing with people with baseball bats and even a samurai sword once. I would also buy drugs, mix them with glucose to dilute them and sell them on and I could make £400 a night, and this is back in the mid 90's. I was also having dealings with a well know motorcycle group (Hells Angels).

I was still having various women here, there, wherever and I'd been married twice by this time. In 1994 I got married for the 3rd time, but was still having women on the side and was drinking far too much. In my life I think I've had sex with around 250 women.

I think sex as a coping mechanism was quite a big thing throughout my life. I used to have a very high sex drive, the more sex I had, the more I needed. With regards to offending, I knew it was wrong; if you've ever seen those cartoons with the devil and an angel on someone's shoulders, with the devil saying *'yeah, go on, you know you want to, you'll enjoy it'*. Well he's pretty big at this time (offending from 2004 till arrest in 2009) and the angel is quiet.

I was ashamed of myself after my last offences, I was drinking more and more and I was well ashamed of myself. When I was charged I pleaded guilty to everything straight away. I thought I'm glad she (victim's therapist) did report me, now I can get something done about it. It was a genuine relief that things could change. My victim's Mother made me promise to do 3 things, take all the help I can find, don't kill myself and make sure I don't do it again! So far, I've kept those promises. Then I went to prison in 2009.

Dave: So Pete, when you went back to prison this time, how was it different from your earlier experiences

Pete: I'd been in prison a lot all of my life and was worried I was going to get life or an IPP. The judge gave me 9 yrs. I eventually get to a therapy prison and there are that many people willing to offer me help, I thought I was on a different planet! I thought, this isn't prison! People were willing to help me better myself. I've been used to people calling me a rotten egg and saying I'd done this and that, but now I was getting help. I also did education and got level 2 numeracy and literacy. I got a lot of help from women and all this help basically turned my thinking around; instead of thinking as women as sex objects, I thought they have got another purpose in life. I did a sharp left in my thinking; I thought women have got a purpose other than as a sexual plaything for me.

I then started on Core Sex Offender Treatment Programme where all of my facilitators were women. I was getting all this help but still wasn't sure why I did it. But the way my thinking has changed has helped me delve inside myself and find out things, and I came to the conclusion I thought of women as sexual objects, no matter what age they were. Now I know that, can understand what I was thinking, I can carry on with my life; I'm still not drinking or taking drugs.

I'd just finished the core and just before release my facilitator approached me and told me about Circles so I thought I'll go for that, my family had disowned me and I had no one outside. I was one of the first Circles in this project.

I thought I'll give it a go. I thought its people I can meet and talk about things with. I was a little bit worried about being judged but I'm thinking, they should know what they are getting into, they signed up for it. It was a bit scary the first time but I thought, get in there. I was open and up front and thought that's how I've got to be.

Dave: Have you ever had that type of help before?

Pete: No! It started in prison where people were willing to help me. All you have to do is ask for help. I'd always tried to sort problems out in the past but if I couldn't succeed I thought sod it!

Dave: What did the Circle help you with, how did they support you?

Pete: Just by being there. They are someone you can have a moan at about what's happened that day; they were there when there was just nobody else. I'd just come out of prison and the world was a strange place, it was a big culture shock and they were there to help me transition from prison back into freedom and helped me along the way. The regular meetings, that structure was very important and I miss it, it was giving me something in the week to do, to look forward to. At first, the meetings were a little too structured with flipcharts, and I thought it's a bit like programmes this [Sex Offender Treatment Programmes; SOTP], asking about sexual thinking and things like that, but I would deal with that at the start of the meeting then it would become more social. One of the volunteer's church group gave me a donation of £50 after he approached them on my behalf, I was able to buy clothes with this money as all I had after release was the clothes I stood up in. I was so grateful for that.

I also remember a time I was trying to get housing and I'd been messed about by the council who wrote to me and said I was not eligible. In the past I would have screwed the letter up and gone to the pub and gone totally wasted, but this time, with the help of the Circle I wrote a letter to them and got a positive reply. I was really happy that a different way of solving problems had worked.

Everything has changed now, I consider other people before myself now, I consider my neighbors, and I try to be polite and helpful. My whole outlook has changed, I'm much more positive and I feel like I'm living a different life now.

With my Circle, regular volunteers would have made it much better. Some of them left the Circle and I would always think is it me? Is it my crime? Is it something I've done? I started to think along those lines after one or two of them left. That's about it though, I enjoyed it. That's why I come back to help you train the new volunteers.

People have gone out of their way to help me and I'm grateful for that, so helping you is my way of giving something back. It makes me feel good to know that I'm helping you to train the new volunteers. Its good and I want to continue doing it for a long time in the future, and maybe one day, be a Circle volunteer

Core member: James
Age at time of interview: 54
Offence history: Taking/making/distributing indecent photographs of children. Attempted rape of female under 16/Indecent assault against male under 14
Circle status: Ongoing weekly meetings
Circle duration: Circle started in October 2016. Sessions to date: 28

I lived with Mum and Dad, a normal family. When I was 10, my Grandma died. That had quite an impact because I blamed my family for that; they switched off the life support machine and at 10 yrs old I didn't understand these things; then I wasn't allowed to go to the funeral and I became anti the family. I didn't really want to have much to do with them. I was close to my aunt, who was probably the closest person to me, apart from my Mum when I was growing up. I played youth club football from 11 to 19 yrs old. I enjoyed junior school, but had problems in secondary school and skipped school for two terms until I got caught.

When I left school, I was a bit lazy and did what I wanted to do, not what others wanted me to do. I wanted to be an electrician but didn't get into college. I was arguing with my Dad, we didn't get on and he asked me to leave, and I slept rough for a few days. I eventually moved back home though.

My first girlfriend was when I was 14 yrs old, but that's what caused the problems with my Dad because I was told not to see her; so of course, being a teenager I did the exact opposite. I eventually found out that her Mum was a prostitute and that was why they didn't want me to see her. They moved away so I borrowed a bicycle and cycled 15 miles to see her, the police were called because I was missing, and they rang my parents to let them know I was OK. That was also my first sexual experience that night, with her. She was a year younger than me, she was 13 yrs old and I was 14 yrs old. I don't really remember that much about the sex, it sort of just happened.

My Dad died in 1983. I was in Ireland and came home, more for my Mum, not my Dad. Looking for work, someone told me about a job in a children's home. I moved there to work and was incredibly lonely. I was offered a job at a school with temporary accommodation and after several months, I met my victim's Mother. My victim went to the school so I knew of her but didn't realise until I got together with her Mum and went to the house. Several months later I committed my first offences against my girlfriend's daughter as well as against one of the boys who lived next door; this was over a period of 18 months.

I decided to leave the area as my girlfriend had met someone else and I was really jealous and just wanted to get away. I then worked for a single Father as a nanny and housekeeper for 6 months. I then got another nanny job, looking after a boy and a girl for 5 yrs then moved to looking after a boy and a girl.

I had no problems getting interviews because I was a male; people were inquisitive as to why I wanted a job. So I got interviews because of this and my references, I didn't have a problem getting work. After another 5 yrs, in 1997 I decided I'd had enough of this; I gave notice to leave in July but was arrested in June.

I was running a football team and there was an allegation from one of the boys. It was dropped, they said because of lack of evidence but I say it's because there was no evidence to find. The contact offences I've done they know about, there's nothing else I've done.

Then in 1999, I got arrested for my previous offences, my victim had come forward and said something. I denied everything, more to myself than anyone else and that made things really difficult. Then they came and asked about the boys next door to my first victim, that's when I was on judges remanded in a hostel. My Mum and sister came to see me on Boxing Day. That's pretty much it until I went to prison and got out in 2004.

Prison was horrible! I didn't know anyone; the guy I shared with was a seasoned criminal who knew the ropes. He made me come out of the cell and that made life a little easier. I was still maintaining my innocence; before the trial though, I told my sister and my Mum that I was guilty, but before that I had to tell myself and that's why it took so long to tell my family. I was protecting myself from what I'd done. My sister was OK on the surface, on this sentence it's different with her because we now speak a lot more now and back then I was more economical with the truth, so there was still some denial.

I did the core SOTP [Sex Offender Treatment Programme]; I found the SOTP very intrusive and a lot of people didn't like talking. I often wondered why what I was being asked was relevant; I also found it hard to trust. I did what I needed to do on the course but that was about it. I didn't volunteer information, I'd answer questions but I didn't go above or beyond.

When I got out I got a place of my own, then my Mum died that first Christmas out. That really hit me! I wasn't close to my brother at all, I didn't speak to my other sister and the sister I did speak to, I wasn't welcome at the house by her husband, so we could only meet outside her house and she had to travel to meet me. That's when things started going downhill, my sister had noticed things were not right with me but she didn't know how to help because I wouldn't talk to her.

Always, throughout that period, I've had an interest in children. It's always been there. I'm exploring this with my probation officer now and she asked me when did I first notice that interest? I've thought about that as I wasn't sure, and on reflection I think even in my teens that interest was there. I know it sounds strange because it was an interest in people my own age back then, which is OK, but I still have that interest as well as an interest in people my own age too.

I got out and got a house in 2005; people knew I was sex offender and it caused a bit of trouble. People found out because of police coming to the house. I was arrested regarding one of the boys of a friend, but again there was nothing there, just some pictures of the boy on his bed in his pants. Looking back they were inappropriate and I accept that now. It was dropped on the day in court, but the friend I had was hostile to me and there was some trouble at the house. The police responded when someone was trying to get into my house, the police then suggested I go to the council to get accommodation. I got a nice flat but was still not good with myself and wasn't working, this was is 2006.

I then started to notice some of the children in the area and used that memory to masturbate to those fantasies then used the internet to find more pictures. Again, I've got no reason to lie now; I only ever went on 'my-space' which is an 18+ site, but the police decided the guy in the image was not 18, and I got done for it. I know it sounds like I trying to minimise it, and that's what they said on SOTP [Sex Offender Treatment

Programme] but I'm just telling the truth. I never had any pornography, videos or anything like that. I knew I had this problem though and I told my sister. I think she had an inkling, she knew I had that interest from my previous crimes. I tried to get help, I asked for help and they said there was no funding, so I got nowhere. But even when I was looking for help I was still offending, I was still looking for pictures and the whole of my sex life at that time was fantasies about children. There were no adult thoughts for a good 18 months prior to going to prison.

Dave: If you'd gotten some help then, maybe some counselling, do you think things would have been different?

James: You know something; I think I would have carried on. The way I was, I think I would have carried on looking because I needed to be in prison to take me out of that situation, I needed to be somewhere where I didn't have that stimulus. Even when they took my computer away before the trial, I bought another laptop, not just to look for pictures but that was a part of it. They said they found pictures on the laptop so there were 2 separate charges; it doesn't matter if it's one charge or a hundred it's just as bad; but I was still defending myself saying I've gone to prison for a few pictures when someone with thousands of pictures gets community service.

I went to prison in 2007. I then withdrew into myself after a massive row with someone, I refused to eat, I threw food at the officers when they tried to get me to eat and it got to the stage where if I'd carried on there would have been serious health issues. One day, a prison officer gave me a really stern talking too and it's what I needed. That's when I decided to tell the SOTP facilitators everything, including what I was thinking inside. The course had evolved slightly and felt less intrusive and I got much more out of it the second time around. The first time on SOTP we just talked about my offence and that was not my problem, the second time I did SOTP we also talked about my thoughts and feelings too.

Dave: How would you say you have problem solved throughout your life James?

James: I buried my head in the sand, that's the only way to describe it, thinking problems would go away. I'm very different now; there has been a massive change; now I may still hope problems will go away or leave things for a little while to see how they go but I don't leave them completely and most things I will face head on. Now I will talk to people, back then I was very much alone even though I had people around me.

It's when I was at open prison I wrote to Circles UK at Reading and asked about Circles. They sent me some information and told me different things. Then through my probation officer I learned about Circles when I got out, I was told there was a waiting list and it may be hard to get onto a Circle, but I then got the news I had a Circle in September.

Dave: What did you think Circles was about?

James: I knew it was for sex offenders, I knew this from a leaflet on my wing. I then checked it out on the internet on one of my town visits so I knew a bit from that. I wasn't quite sure what was involved with it, if I'm honest, I thought it would be more us and them because it was going through probation and the prison so at first I thought it's just another organisation tacked onto them but its more informal, so I still had the attitude if it happens great, if not then no problem. Talking to my probation officer after release I felt that it would be nice to meet up with someone different because that's what I needed, I didn't really know anyone outside. I still, even now count them as more as professionals than friends because they are not friends with you, but then they are not professional either, it's like something in between. I just see them as people, not paid or volunteers. Thinking about it, if they were paid you may wonder are they really interested in me or is it just a job to them? So being a volunteer does sound better. When you are a volunteer you are giving up your time and people seem to appreciate that more than maybe someone who is paid, although lots of people who are paid to help people do that not for the money but because it's what they want to do. It's not just a job for them.

From my perspective as a Core Member, being volunteers is a lot better. It's like meeting someone, a friend who you are getting to know as you go along, but knowing that one day it will end and that's the sad part of it I guess. Because it will end there does have to be that professional line drawn which is sad in one way because you do get to know people. But that's the same in all walks of life, you meet people and you move on.

Dave: How important is having the structure of a regular meeting?

James: The structure is not important to me, the meeting is important but sometimes, on occasion, I could have done without having a meeting at that time on that day because I wanted to do other things and I've had to put things off to accommodate the Circles meeting. But then, it's not just me, we're trying to get 5 people together here. Sometimes I think an hour is not enough, when we went for the meal there was no set time but it took longer, so maybe a little bit more flexibility on time may be good but again; that may be difficult of the volunteers because they have to commit their time, they also have to travel.

Maybe also have more than one meeting a week as an option, have your set meeting but then have an optional meeting at stressful times.

Dave: How else could Circles be improved?

James: In my own experience it's served the purpose from a social side, with my Circle it's been difficult on a practical side because the one time I needed help they couldn't help. I was moving flats and could have used some help, but there were issues with insurance and health and safety, things like that, so they couldn't help me move. Also, meetings being cancelled at the last minute for issues with the volunteers like illness, this can be troublesome when I'm trying to plan my day, and you get left in limbo.

Dave: What have you gotten out of the Circle James?

James: I've learned to talk to people, so it's been good to be able to come and talk to them and not have any worries that they will go blabbing off to someone. It's nice to be able to talk to people in a relaxed atmosphere, I've also never been judged by the volunteers and I've found I can ask them questions as well. I remember having a meeting in a coffee house and we were talking, and I asked them why do you want to work with people like me, why do you do this? I think they were a bit taken a back but they did answer and it was refreshing to hear how people want to help people and to understand why people have done what they have done; it's good that there are people who do want to help.

It's nice to be able to discuss things with my Circle, I can tell them things without holding back. If I do say something, they don't just listen; they ask questions, they probe. They don't just say 'oh right' and that's it, they ask questions to find what's behind the problem.

I've certainly got that from the Circle; that I can talk to people and don't have to worry about what I say. However, I'm not quite sure about the minutes that are written after the session. I feel the Core Members should be able to see them as that would build trust; again it's like when you have MAPPA meetings. I'm not involved and I know they are talking about me; my probation officer says it's all good because you're doing so well but it can't be all good. If I could see the minutes it would help to minimise that 'them and us' attitude.

Overall though, it's been very good for me. You've got me out to a different location, I've got to meet people, there are more people I can talk to. So even something as simple as when I change my phone and have to text people my new number, instead of sending to two or three people, I have several to send to now, same with happy New Year's messages. It may seem a small thing but it's not. That contact matters.

A Volunteers Perspective

Volunteer: Kate
Age at time of interview: 68
Occupation: Retired probation officer/minister
Circle status: Currently on a Circle that started in October 2015, meeting bi-weekly
Circle duration: To date: 20 months/52 sessions.

I go back right to the very beginning of Circles in this country. When restorative justice first came in, the Quakers were very involved with it and I was ministering at that time. I heard about it then and dipped my toe in the water, my background was probation and I studied criminology before that. I didn't have time to volunteer but kept an interest in what was happening in the criminal justice system and restorative justice. When I retired and had more time, I thought it was time to become involved; got in touch with Circles and ended up as a volunteer with them. The Circle only lasted 3 months because the Core Member moved away, but it was a very useful experience. There was a lot that was good, but there was also a lot that I would criticise about that particular set up.

And then I moved areas. Before I left I spoke to my coordinator and asked what was going on up here and I got in touch with the project in the new area and it went in from there.

I was retired so I had more time on my hands. For the last 20 years I've been in Christian ministry so it's a natural part of me to want to give something to the community and to do something with the time I had. I felt that any retired priest can help with church services, but not any retired priest could do this sort of work, work that my background and experience helps me to do.

People who commit sexual offences are today's outsiders; and from a Christian perspective, outsiders are the people to be bought inside and of all the outcasts and outsiders I would say that those who have committed sexual offences are pretty much on the bottom of that list.

The papers don't help either. I think everyone wants, psychologically, to focus our negatives on someone we can think of as worse than ourselves. You only have to look at high profile sex offence court cases. You can see the members of the public out there, storming to get into the court or throwing bricks at the prison van holding the accused; there does seem to be something within human kind to find someone to let their aggression out on! Offenders appear to be on the receiving end of that aggression, and if you look at the different categories of offender, sexual offenders seem to be thought of as the worst, especially offences against children.

I thought the training for the SLF's Circles was good; I do think it could have majored more on the need for the volunteer's commitment to the role. There is a lack of balance between males and females, young and old but that is not a fault of Circles. I think it's inevitable that there will be a high rate of students who are studying criminology, psychology, that sort of thing; but the trouble is for that group, even for the most committed their life situation is such that when university comes to an end they have to get a job, or they move back home, or they have interviews to attend and then they are not in control of what their hours will be, this impacts on their ability to make Circles meetings.

I was however, very encouraged on the training day was that I would not be asked to work with a Core Member who had a learning disability. I feel that I work with a very verbal and intellectual approach, so I was very gratified to learn that I would not be asked to work with someone I did not feel I would be able to; there was no pressure to work with a Core Member I didn't want to and that was great and exactly the right way to go.

In our Circle, we have developed a good relationship between all of us, we do communicate with each other and the Core Member is just a super Core Member to have. I was really frustrated with how the Core Member was dealt with by the criminal justice system towards the end of his time in prison, it was just outrageous! If we're going to work really well with someone you need to have an idea of when he is going to be discharged, so that you can, at the right time start preparing for his release. You can't do this months before he is released because you'll be setting them up for frustration. So we thought we knew he was being released, everyone said this was so, and we worked with him towards him getting out. He is a very positive person and we started preparing him for release, he engages well with us and works hard to look at getting ready for life on the outside; we then hear that his parole date has been put back several months. We then had to stop preparing him and the Circle just became social chit chat. OK, the Core Member still enjoyed the meetings and you could say that our relationship grew but I found that very frustrating. Then we got the news that he was getting his parole so we think we can start again preparing him for release, but it was only 2 weeks later that he was released and this was before we had properly prepared him for life outside after over a decade in prison.

Also, we knew he needed identification; he didn't have a birth certificate or any photo I.D. and the prison system did not allow for him to use his own prison photo to help him get some I.D. Sure enough, post release, the lack of photo I.D. did become an issue and did contribute to delays in him getting the simple things like a free bus pass or a bank account. Finally, when released, he was put in a taxi and then told he had to make his own way from the prison to the hostel; he's been in prison for over a decade, was in his 70's and was not that physically fit.

Dave: Bearing these things in mind Kate, what positives have you personally taken from working with your Core Member on his Circle?

Kate: It's a very useful and important task and I think without the Circle he may have thought of breaking his license conditions to get back into prison as I do feel he's been very institutionalised, even at the hostel, that's still like a little institution for him. He's still going out on the bus to different places but I think it's still quite an institutionalised existence.

When this Circle ends, I think it will be a very mixed feeling. Once he's settled into his own, permanent accommodation I feel that we will have done all we can do and it will be time to move onto another Circle. It might be frustrating because we may have to end the Circle before its ideal; because of all the delays he had he's still not in his own accommodation; I certainly hope there may be some flexibility when we end the Circle, and if we could extend the Circle to support him for a while when he moves into his own place then that would be better. As a person I quite like things that have a beginning, middle and end, and my temperament likes things that have a comparatively short time frame. I don't like open ended arrangements and that why I found it so frustrating waiting for his parole date, with no end in sight. So in a way, I'm quite looking forward to the Circle ending, it will feel the right thing to be doing at that time.

I would encourage anyone who is thinking about volunteering on a Circle; it's highly satisfying but I would want to stress the commitment needed. The men we are dealing with have undergone an awful lot of rejection, so it's important that that the volunteers regularly turn up to meetings as the Core Member's may take it really personally if they don't. However, I will do another Circle after this one has ended, you can be sure of that!

Coordinators Perspective

I have been working within the prison system for 27 years since 1989, and I started first as an instructor in the woodmill at HMP Ranby. Here, I helped to train prisoners to work machines that produced furniture for cells and offices within prisons, as well as outside contracts. This is where I first became aware of the positive effect on the prisoners that giving them responsibility and a structure to their day had. Men that had never worked before in their lives, found a pride and satisfaction in doing a good job and being responsible for a machine, and I know of plenty who found work after release based on the experience they had received in Ranby's woodmill.

After 15 years at Ranby I decided on a change of career and made my mind up to become a prison officer. I went to look at HMP Whatton and during the tour I was given a talk on SOTP [Sex Offender Treatment Progamme]. Well, for the first time in my life a light bulb went off in my head and I thought, that's what I want to do. I passed all of the tests and started as an officer facilitator at Whatton in 2006. In the next 10 years, I trained for and delivered all of the programmes that we ran, particularly enjoying the challenge of working with high risk men. However, I began to notice that although the men received lots of support and help in Whatton to manage their risks, after release there was next to no support especially for high risk men released without family or friends' support. These men were often released into a new area, their families and friends had deserted them and they had almost always lost their jobs; all of this as a consequence of their offending. I began to think that all these men needed was somewhere they could go, once a week where they could meet people who knew them and their risks. That way they could get some support with managing their risks and they would have a better chance at keeping safe and not reoffending.

Then came Circles! I role played for one of their early trainings sessions and was immediately hooked into the premise (this was the second light bulb moment of my life). This was what I had been thinking about and I wanted to be a part of it. I decided to apply for the position of coordinator for the community Circles and have now been in post for 17 months. It's still the most challenging, rewarding and worthwhile job I've ever had, or ever will have.

There are challenges of course, it's difficult to get volunteers together at the same time and place to start a Circle, and the Core Members have their own issues that come with being at high or very high risk of reoffending. Another challenge often faced, and touched upon by Kate in her interview, is the difficulty that Core Members face when dealing with the very real frustrations that being released into the community can bring. Finding accommodation, organizing benefits, even obtaining a bank account can be challenges that the Core Member could find difficult to navigate without the help of a Circle. Volunteers can also be frustrated by these challenges, but they should be seen as a reason for the Circle's existence, rather than a barrier to the Circle working.

However, despite the challenges, I love the autonomy and creativity that the role allows, and when you see a Core Member really interacting pro socially with his Circle, talking about how he is managing his risk, moving into follow on accommodation, finding a job or successfully completing his license period, then that brings huge rewards for the volunteers and myself as well as a feeling of pride. As well as helping some of the most excluded and rejected members of society to reintegrate, we are also actively preventing sexual abuse. Therefore we are preventing further victims and this is the prime reason for a Circle, and something we never lose sight of.

There have been one or two Core Members who have been recalled for breaking licence conditions (although to date, no Core Member has sexually reoffended) and some have left early of their own accord against the wishes of the Circle, probation and the MOSOVO unit (Management of Sexual Offenders and Violent Offenders) but they are exceptions and we always remind the volunteers that the Core Members are accountable for their own actions.

Conclusion

During the interviews presented in this chapter, I was struck by the enthusiasm of the Core Members to undertake any work which could help the SLF and our CoSA. Several Core Members regularly help us by attending out initial training session; there they talk to the volunteers about what a Circle is, what it means to them and how important the commitment is. I was also interested to see just how important the 'small' things are; having people to text 'happy new year' to, having someone to listen to you if you've had a bad day, getting help to write a letter or having a coffee with people who are there because they want to be. These things that we can take for granted mean the world to a Core Member.

I was also struck by how often we hear about avoidant or inappropriate coping methods that the majority of Core Members' practice throughout their lives, as well as their willingness to talk candidly to the volunteers about their sexual thinking. Having 'normal' members of the public listen to them without judging them, shows the Core Members that there are people that will help, that won't define them by just their offending actions, but will look for potential in every one of them.

Having a Circle is not an easy ride for the Core Members, and there are learning points for all Circles projects, for example—more flexibility (where possible) with the time and duration of meetings.

These interviews show that the Core Members and volunteers get a great deal out of their time on a Circle; for the Core Member it teaches them that people can and will give them a second chance, and that they are worth something as people. This increase in self-worth and self-belief, in itself, can be enough to move them away from reoffending. For the volunteers, they get a deep sense of satisfaction from helping a vulnerable person rebuild an offence free life; I often tell them that they could literally be saving a life, and this fact resonates deeply with them.

I believe that CoSA is of incredible importance to our society. We prevent further victims, we help rehabilitate and reintegrate back into society some of the most marginalised, misunderstood and hated members of society and we also work to help to change public perceptions of our client group. One day, I hope that those convicted of sexual offences can be helped and worked with openly, calmly, rationally and with the understanding from communities that if they come together to help support those who have sexually offended, then they will actively be helping to prevent another victim.

Reference

Hanvey, S., Philpot, T., & Wilson, C. (2011). *A community-based approach to the reduction of sexual reoffending*. London: Jessica Kingsley.

8

Future Directions: Alternative Circles of Support and Accountability Models and Minority Groups

Kerensa Hocken, Claire Good, Helen Elliott, Carrie Webb, Helen O'Connor, and Kim Cox

Introduction

This chapter is split into two sections. The first will focus on the different models of Circles of Support and Accountability (CoSA), some already introduced around the world and others are theoretically driven considerations of how the CoSA model could be shaped. This

K. Hocken (✉)
HMPPS Whatton, Whatton, UK

C. Good
Safer Living Foundation, Visits Centre, Nottingham, UK

H. Elliott
Bishop Grosseteste University, Lincoln, UK

C. Webb
Circles South East, Didcot, Oxford, UK

H. O'Connor • K. Cox
HMPPS Midlands Psychology Service, Whatton, Nottingham, UK

H. Elliott et al. (eds.), *Sexual Crime and Circles of Support and Accountability*, Sexual Crime, https://doi.org/10.1007/978-3-319-74823-8_8

includes considering psychologically informed Circles, specifically focusing on the attachment needs of individuals convicted of sexual crime as well as Circles for non-offending individuals in the community who are concerned about their sexual thoughts or behaviour. These models will be discussed in conjunction with theory and empirical findings that support their foundations. Part two of this chapter will explore how CoSA can work for certain minority groups, including CoSA for transgender populations, deaf individuals and young people. Discussion of how the Circle might look, client specific considerations and volunteer selection and training necessary for working with these groups will be explored. Finally, some conclusions will be drawn about the future of CoSA.

Different Models of CoSA

A Case for Psychologically Informed Circles

One of the core functions of a Circle is social support: someone who the Core Member can talk about their problems with, seek advice or guidance from, try out new social activities with, and importantly knowing there is someone who cares about them. These are all vital functions for humans; as a social animal we are neurologically designed to live in social groups and as such we have a well-developed capacity for attachment to others. Our attachment abilities enable us to bond with care givers as babies and to be fearful of strangers, enable us to nurture our young, to have trusting and caring relationships with people outside of our immediate kin network, and of course they allow us to develop and maintain long lasting romantic attachments. These human abilities have evolved in order to help us survive as a species and as such our attachment instincts are important for survival. Given our biological predisposition for living in social groups, rejection can be one of the biggest triggers to feeling threatened, resulting in feelings of fear, anxiety, anger and shame. In fact, research shows that loneliness can increase mortality to such an extent it is comparable with other accepted risk factors for mortality such as smoking (Holt-Lunstad, Smith, Baker, Harris, & Stephenson, 2015).

The impact of social isolation on reintegration and risk for reoffending for people who have sexual convictions is well recognised (Blake & Gannon, 2011; Marshall, 2010; Ward, Keenan, & Hudson, 2000) and is indeed the key impetus for the CoSA project. It seems then that a core function of a Circle appeals to a fundamental human need for affiliation with others and the provision of a Circle of Support for people with sexual convictions may be enhanced if volunteers are aware of and responsive to the individual attachment needs of the Core Member.

For people who have a disrupted attachment history—a characteristic of many CoSA clients, the attachment capabilities are also disrupted, resulting in a lack of understanding about how to build trust with others and in some cases, a deep discomfort at receiving kindness and support from others (Glibert, 2009). Thus they may find it difficult to respond to and benefit from the support offered in a Circle. Having an understanding of this and being able to respond in a psychologically informed way to these difficulties when running a Circle is likely to offer the best chance of success, helping the Core Member to relate to others in a functional way. This does not require Circles' sessions to be 'therapy', or go beyond the remit of CoSA volunteers' abilities, but it allows the Circle to engage in activities which help to get the best from the exprience. The case of Dave below shows some of the social difficulties Core Members experience due to disrupted attachment and the simple changes psychologically informed volunteers could make.

Case of Dave

Dave has a disrupted attachment history, being raised in care from the age of 7 after being removed from his parents due to safeguarding concerns. As an adult, he is not close to his parents and has no close friends. Dave feels threatened by eye contact from others because he has not learnt to feel safe in relationships. Although he is able to sit in a group for a formal meeting, this triggers his anxiety, which he masks by pretending to find the discussions boring and not sharing his inner thoughts or vulnerabilities. In recognition of this, the Circle began to do activities with him that removed the need for direct prolonged eye contact and face to face interaction, such as cooking. During the first session of cooking with the Circle, Dave was visibly more relaxed and engaged, he also opened up about his previous life experiences and talked for the first time about his own relationship with his parents.

The concept of psychologically informed rehabilitative efforts have been recognised as important in enhancing rehabilitation opportunities for those in the criminal justice system. For example, the Enabling Environments award offered by the Royal Collage of Psychiatrists recognise environments that promote positive relationships, a sense of belonging, growth and welling being for clients. Similarly, Psychologically Informed Planned Environments (PIPES) for people in the criminal justice system with personality disorder have also been recognised as beneficial in engaging clients and improving rehabilitation outcomes through better relationships. These benefits clearly map onto the aims of CoSA. Thus having coordinators trained in attachment and offering supervision to volunteers could provide the necessary knowledge base to enable Circles to become 'psychologically informed'.

CoSA Volunteers with Previous Sexual Offences

The rehabilitative impact of receiving and providing peer support shows promising results in the substance misuse fields (Tracy & Wallace, 2016) and has been reasonably well documented in prisons, especially in the context of therapeutic communities (Stevens, 2012). Until recently, very little has been documented about these benefits for people convicted of sexual offences. It is possible that the peer support method has been discounted as being unsuitable for this group due to the belief it will encourage offending through allowing paedophilic networking. However in a unique exploration of this area Perrin, Blagden, Winder and Dillon (2017) reported that men convicted of sexual offences in prison in peer-support roles did seem to gain rehabilitative benefit. Specifically, the experiences of 'doing good' and 'giving back' allowed them to adopt a non-offending, prosocial identity. The authors suggest that this allows a parallel move away from the offender identity; something which research proposes is likely to facilitate desistance (Maruna, 2001). This raises the question as to whether having volunteers with sexual convictions on a Circle may also bring rehabilitative benefits for the Core Member and volunteer. This is not a model that has ever been reported, according to the authors' knowledge and represents a bold move. However, providing the process is carefully managed, it is one that could be considered. Certain safeguards may be necessary such as ensuring that the convicted volunteer has completed any treatment and punishment sentences and neither they or the Core Member have engaged in offending related to networking. The Core Member and other volunteers would also need to consent. The case study below is written by Peter, someone with a sexual conviction who feels that the opportunity to have a sexually convicted CoSA volunteer would be beneficial to rehabilitation.

A Service User's Perspective

My name is Peter and I was convicted for committing a sexual offence in 2010. I believe there is great benefit in using peer mentors as volunteers in the rehabilitation of people with sexual convictions. This technique has been used successfully in the areas of drug, alcohol and gambling addiction and support groups for depression and anxiety. Peer mentoring in prisons has also proved highly effective. For myself this would give me a purpose in life. To be able to do something meaningful to help others who struggle, as I have done in the past, to control unwanted thoughts and feelings. I feel that if I could help somebody else to avoid creating any more victims, then this would in some small way compensate for some of the damage I have done in the past.

Serving the community in this way would enable me to make use of some of the techniques that have helped me to cope, and in helping others this would help me to bring something good out of the bad of my past behaviour. Using my skills and knowledge to help others in this way would also mean there were a lot more people I really did not want to let down and this would help to strengthen my own defences to help me avoid creating any further victims. Helping others is very beneficial to self-esteem and strengthens empathy and compassion which are strong factors in avoiding offending.

To meet and talk with somebody who has been where you are and understands the difficulties you are facing, but can demonstrate that it is possible to get past these problems and construct a worthwhile life without harming others, is very encouraging. This arguably has greater power than advice from people who have never faced these struggles. Support from somebody for whom the problems are real is a huge help to people who are struggling and helps to give us purpose and focus and something to aspire towards. Many of us have never had encouragement or seen possibility of success and genuine recovery and seeing this for real can make a big difference to people.

Peter's words illustrate the rehabilitative benefits that volunteering with CoSA could have for both Core Member and volunteer. Adopting this model would increase the number of people one Circle is able to help and would also provide opportunities for suitable successful Core Members to in turn assist others.

A Preventative Approach to Circles

Crime prevention is becoming the buzzword within the criminal justice system, with the surge for preventative efforts now stronger than ever. The history of preventative efforts stretches back to the 1980s/90s when the first real attempts to prevent crime were made. However, these preventative efforts were different to the ones proposed now, as the main goals were to ensure the benefits of crime did not outweigh costs, and that communities would actively work to counter the threat of crime to reduce the chances of themselves becoming a victim (Crawford & Evans, 2016). This led to a focus on policing, to make crime difficult to commit without detection, making societies safer. However, with limited resources and an extremely complex and difficult task on their hands, prevention became secondary to the main task of policing—to detect, arrest and prosecute (Crawford & Evans, 2016). Since, things have moved on and there is a much heavier focus on social crime prevention, looking at the root causes of crime and social influences. This led to a movement towards reducing motivation to offend by looking at the social influences that increase crime for individuals (developmental prevention; Farrington, 2007; McAra & McVie, 2012), and exploring the role community can play in crime prevention.

Despite this movement towards prevention, in the UK, the criminal justice system's response to sexual crime remains solely reactive, only dealing with the problem of sexual offences once they have been committed and a victim(s) has been created. This is not true of other countries, for example in 2005 Germany introduced Prevention Project Dunkelfeld—a revolutionary movement towards safer communities, through providing free treatment to individuals in the community concerned about their sexual thoughts or behaviour. Via Prevention Project Dunkelfeld, people living in the community who fear they may offend against children can take part in preventative treatment programmes. Recruitment is assisted by mass media campaigns that utilise billboards and television to convey empathy and minimise discrimination and shame. In line with these objectives, the billboards and television campaigns quote the following: "Do you like children more than you/they like? You are not guilty because of your sexual desire, but you are responsible for your sexual behaviour. There is help! Don't be an offender!".

This progressive approach to dealing with sexual crime and making communities safer has been shown to be successful in Germany, raising the question of how CoSA could adopt a preventative approach to its programme. At present, CoSA are only available to those who are known to the criminal justice system for their involvement in a sexual crime. But, what if we were to offer CoSA to those who were not known to the criminal justice system? Research estimates the prevalence of paedophilia is between 3 and 5% in the general population (Seto, 2008). However, whilst such statistical research is available and ongoing, only few offences are accounted for by official statistics and a significant number of cases are never reported to the authorities. This suggests that a significant proportion of child sexual abuse is ongoing and will not be detected. It also the case that there are a number of people in the general population who fear they may offend against children, but have not yet done so. Organisations such as 'Virped' (an online forum for those attracted to children who do not want to offend) demonstrate this, with almost 2000 active members.

With the current system doing minimal to help potential abusers who want to address their risky sexual preferences, CoSA could offer a community attempt to help these individuals and prevent sexual crime. Specific protocols would need to be in place, for example outlining reporting rules and making limits to confidentiality clear. Moreover, identifying 'what works' for this group of non-offending individuals would be imperative, so as not to cause more harm than good. Cantor and McPhail (2016) suggest a number of appropriate treatment targets for this group, based on current (although limited) literature. One of the key suggestions is addressing the issue of stigma around sexual crime. Stigma within sexual minority groups is linked to distress and fear of rejection (Hatzenbuehler, 2009; Liao, Kashubeck-West, Weng, & Deitz, 2015) which can in turn cause shame, anxiety, emotional dysregulation and interpersonal issues. Addressing stigma is a key element of CoSA, with the ethos being to treat Core Members as human beings, and not define them by their previous actions, making this element of the CoSA initiative suited to this group in the community. Moreover, literature suggests that applying some of the psychologically meaningful risk factors for forensic populations to non-offending samples may prove useful. One of the key factors leading to risk of sexual offending is acute vulnerability and loneliness (Cantor, 2014). Thus working with this experience of loneliness and providing a support network for non-offending individuals, another key aspect of CoSA, seems relevant. Lastly, addressing the issue of sexual arousal and preoccupation in some non-offending individuals will be relevant and key to reducing risk of offending, due to the strong association these factors have with committing sexual offences against children (in forensic populations, Mann, Hanson, & Thornton, 2010; McPhail et al., 2017). CoSA plays some role in this, where open discussions are had about sexual thoughts and behaviours, however additional intervention may be necessary, depending on the level of hypersexuality or sexual preoccupation. This may take the form of medication to manage sexual arousal for example (see Winder, Lievesley, Elliott, Hocken, Faulkner, Norman & Kaul, 2017).

With evidence demonstrating the efficacy of preventative treatment programmes for community samples of non-offending individuals (for example Dunkelfeld; Beier et al., 2009), and the knowledge that there are individuals in the community struggling to control their sexual thoughts and behaviour who want help with this, it seems that CoSA could offer a preventative service to support these individuals to not offend. Not only would this provide support to a group of individuals inwardly struggling with very difficult and stigmatised feelings in the community, it would work towards preventing victims of sexual abuse—the ultimate aim of any preventative initiative.

Prison-Based Circles

A final model that must be mentioned is prison-based CoSA. This approach aims to address the issues that are exacerbated for those convicted of sexual offences in the lead up to, and on release from prison, into the community. The prison-CoSA model commences support for Core Members whilst they are still in prison, and continues this during the difficult period of release and once resettling into the community. The model is discussed in detail in Chap. 4 of this book.

CoSA for the Minority

Providing fair access to CoSA for individuals from minority groups is an important human rights issue. The move towards the inclusion of people from groups with protected characteristics (such as those to do with disability or gender) over recent years has resulted in legal requirements to provide them equal access to services and opportunities and requiring that reasonable adjustments be made to facilitate this (Disability Discrimination Act, 1995 & 2005; Equality Act, 2010). These laws also apply to people within the criminal justice system and, in 2010, a prisoner with intellectual disability won a judicial review to have equal access to treatment programmes for violent offending behaviour (Gill v Secretary of State for Justice, 2010). However, in the requirement to make services available for those with protected characteristics, it is important that we do not assume a 'one size fits all' perspective and make only the necessary 'reasonable adjustments' so the service can simply be accessed. It is vital that available services are also suitable and effective for the people that need them.

In this section, we discuss client specific considerations for some minority groups, as well as recommendations for volunteer selection and training, any adaptions that may be needed to the overall CoSA model and report any initial outcomes from Circles already working with these client groups.

Young People with Harmful Sexual Behaviour

Harmful sexual behaviour (HSB) amongst young people is defined as "One or more children engaging in sexual discussions or acts that are inappropriate for their age or stage of development. These can range from using sexually explicit words and phrases to full penetrative sex with other children or adults" (Rich, 2011).

"Retrospective studies present a broad consensus that between 23–40% of all alleged sexual abuse of children and young people is perpetrated by other young people" (NSPCC, 2011). Young People displaying harmful sexual behaviour are a diverse and vulnerable group with many having been abused or neglected themselves. One of the largest research studies into the profile of children and young people displaying HSB in the UK was carried out by Hackett, Phillips, Masson and Balfe in 2013 (Hackett et al., 2013). This research found that of the 700 children and young people they investigated, all of whom had been referred to one of nine UK HSB services:

- the vast majority were white males and the most common age at referral was 15 years;
- around one third were looked after in local authority care;
- two-thirds had experienced trauma or abuse of at least one kind—including physical abuse, emotional abuse, sexual abuse, severe neglect, parental rejection, family breakdown and conflict, domestic violence, parental drug and alcohol abuse;
- specifically, 50% of the young males were found to have been, or were suspected of having been, sexually abused.

Other studies also suggest that young people presenting with HSB commonly have social skills deficits, a lack of sexual knowledge and high levels of social anxiety (Righthand & Welch, 2001; Veneziano & Veneziano, 2002).

In addition to personal characteristics, any sexual abuse or harmful sexual behaviour provokes powerful responses within communities and society, potentially resulting in these young people being labelled for their behaviour. This can cause or further enhance an individual's social isolation and emotional loneliness—key factors that increase risk of reoffending (Cantor, 2014).

Client Specific Considerations

Encouraging young people to engage in CoSA is likely to be more problematic than encouraging an adult to engage. Working closely with partner agencies and potential referring agencies is essential to ensure they fully understand the role of CoSA and how it can benefit young people. To run Young People's Circles successfully, it is vital that the young person and their parent/carer (if appropriate) are motivated to engage, as the Circle can only be undertaken on a voluntary basis with the informed consent of both the young person and their parent/carer. A Young Person's Circle should not be attached to any court order, community sentence plan or licence conditions and enforcement action for non-compliance should not be undertaken.

The engagement of the family is another key difference between Young People's Circles and the adult Circles model. As outlined by the Department for Children, Schools and Families (2009), "families in whatever form they take, are the bedrock of our society. Mothers, fathers, brothers, sisters, grandparents, step family and extended family members provide the support, safety and encouragement in which children grow up and use as a springboard for creating their place within the world. Often it is the commitment of mothers and fathers to do best for their children which motivates the family to overcome the challenges which life throws at them". Young People's Circles should try wherever possible to engage with the family. Parents/Carers can be invited to each Circle Review to talk through changes they have witnessed in relation to the young person. Where these are positive changes, having these acknowledged by both the Circle and the Parents/carers can have a significant positive effect on the young person.

Given the nature of the young people likely to be participating in Young People's Circles, and the research which overwhelmingly shows that a large proportion of those young people who commit sexual offences are likely to have been victims of abuse or neglect themselves, Young People's Circles projects must anticipate that young people may disclose to their Circle previous abuse or neglect. It is for this reason that it is essential volunteers undertake comprehensive safeguarding training so they feel confident they could act appropriately should this situation arise.

The Model

Based on the research outlined, it would seem that there is a very real need for CoSA for Young People. Young People's CoSA would aim to address social isolation, emotional loneliness, social skills deficits and social anxiety by working with these young people before they become an "adult sex offender" with multiple victims. Children and adolescents are still developing, both physically and psychologically, so well-targeted early interventions such as this can be extremely effective in terms of changing recidivist attitudes and behaviour, and so, preventing more victims.

In addition, Circles can be beneficial for young people displaying HSB before they reach the criminal justice system, as well as for those who have already received a caution or conviction for a sexual offence. This is in contrast to adult CoSA, which are only used following an individual's release from custody (apart from the prison-based model at HMP Whatton, as outlined in Chap. 4).

Effective interventions with children and young people with HSB should be holistic and focus on both the specific offence related work as well as wider aspects of the young person's functioning (Hackett, 2014). Young People's Circles can therefore add value to other interventions, by focusing on the wider aspects of young people's functioning such as social skills.

Circles are based within the theoretical framework of the 'Good Lives Model' (GLM) and Young People's Circle are no different. The GLM is a strength based approach to Offender Rehabilitation (Ward & Stewart, 2003). Volunteers will deliver a pro-social intervention building on the young person's strengths, interests and hobbies to ensure the safe inclusion and integration of these young people into the community and reduce chances of social isolation, emotional loneliness and reoffending. The intervention provided by volunteers on a Young People's Circle is likely to be much more practical and creative than the intervention provided on an adult Circle. Young people will typically find it difficult or awkward to engage with a group of 3–5 adults and specifically talking about relationships and sexual behaviour is unlikely to come easy to them. It is therefore important to develop creative ways of getting young people to engage with the Circle and to start talking about these sensitive topics over time (see Fig. 8.1).

It is important to remember that Young People's Circles is not a treatment model, but a supportive one, which aims to reduce the risks of offending by reducing levels of social isolation and emotional loneliness. Therefore although there will be some focus and discussions around sex and relationships, a large amount of the work will involve supporting the young person to develop as a person and increase their protective factors. Types of intervention may therefore include:

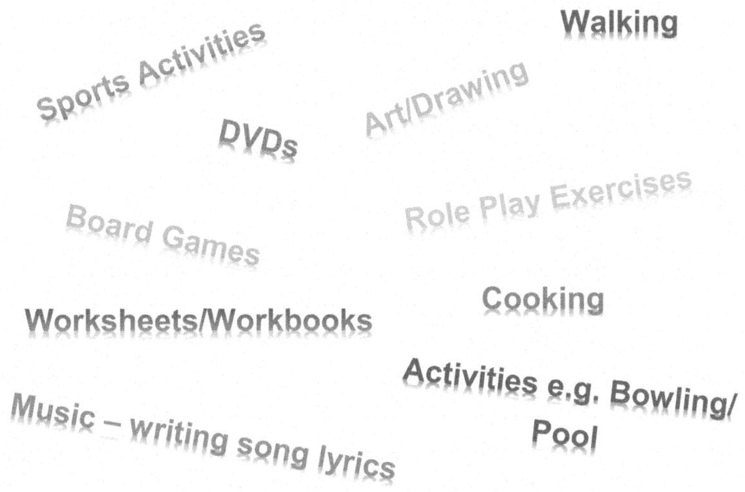

Fig. 8.1 Creative tools to help young people engage with a circle

- Help with independent living skills for example cooking, budgeting, shopping etc.;
- Support with CV writing;
- Help with work experience or volunteering;
- Helping finding work;
- Helping young person to navigate around a local area;
- Introducing young person to positive activities in their local area;
- Accompanying young person to local activities;
- Discussions around sex and positive relationships;
- Talking to young people about appropriate disclosures.

Volunteers should be given a level of autonomy to be creative and come up with creative ways to work with the young person based on their interests.

Volunteer Selection and Training

Appropriate volunteer selection and training is vital to the success of Young People's Circles. All volunteers should go through the same 'safe recruitment' processes as they would for adult Circles. This includes the same core training that is expected for adult Circles. However, in addition, volunteers who wish to work on Young People's Circles will require additional training around the following key areas:

- the role of young people's Circles;
- how young people's Circles will operate;
- an introduction to the youth justice system;
- child protection and safeguarding;
- child and adolescent development and attachment theory;
- how to work effectively with young people.

As with adult Circles, all volunteers will have to complete an enhanced DBS check with the additional check that they do not appear on the barred list of individuals who are unsuitable for working with children.

Once volunteers have been successfully interviewed and trained it is important that they are appropriately matched to a young person. Ideally volunteers would live in the same local community as the young person as this means they have a good local knowledge of the area and the facilities and opportunities available. Each Circle would have between three and five volunteers and these volunteers should be made up of a mix of demographics (age, gender and ethnicity). It is also ideal if the interests of the volunteers could be matched to the interests of the young person so as to help enthuse the young person.

Outcomes

The overall aims of Young People's Circles are:

- reduced (re)offending;
- improved mental health (reduced emotional loneliness);
- increased social integration into the community (leading to increased self-esteem and confidence);
- increased participation in community activities or organisation;
- changes in attitudes towards more social and less criminal attitudes.

Intellectual Disability and Autistic Spectrum Conditions

People with intellectual disability (ID) and Autistic Spectrum Conditions (ASC) are over represented in sexually convicted populations (Guay, Ouimet & Proulx, 2004) and due to their disabilities and the circumstances associated with it, are perhaps in greater need of the support a Circle can offer. When properly adapted for their needs, people with ASC and ID can draw significant benefit from a Circle. It is therefore crucial that all Circles projects consider the feasibility of offering Circles to this client group so that equality of access is provided.

Client Specific Considerations

Intellectual Disability and Autistic Spectrum Conditions are neurodevelopmental disorders, which means they are disorders where there is an impairment of the growth and development of the brain, usually in evidence from childhood. The impairment can cause deficits in various areas of the individuals functioning such as occupational, social, and academic domains. ID is typically diagnosed where there are deficits in the social, practical and conceptual (usually an IQ below 70) domains of functioning. ASC is diagnosed where there are deficits in the social and communication domains.

Research has found a general trend that individuals with ID and ASC are over-represented in sexual offending populations; for example, in young people who show sexually harmful behaviour, it is estimated that approximately one third to one half have ID or significant learning difficulties (Almond, Canter, & Salfati, 2006) and Mouridsen (2012) suggests that sexual offences are more common than other types of crime committed by people with ASC.

In the UK, approximately 10% of prisoners who complete sexual offending treatment programmes have ID or borderline IQ (NOMS, personal communication, 22 December, 2013) compared to a prevalence of 1–3% in the general population for ID (Volkmar & Dykens, 2002; Maulik, Mascarenhas, Mathers, Dua, & Saxena, 2011). This illustrates that a significant proportion of people with sexual convictions will have ID and ASC, and thus may be one of the many referred for CoSA.

The unique psychological and social circumstances associated with having ID or ASC suggest that these groups may in fact have a greater need for the support a Circle can offer. They are less likely to have a close social support networks and more likley to have relationship problems (Lindsay et al. 2006), more likely to be open to the influence of others due to increased suggestibility (Gudjonsson & Clare, 1995), less able to independently access, use and benefit from community resources such as public transport, benefits and leisure services (Matson, Rivet, Fodstad, Dempsey, & Boisjoli, 2009), more likely to be unemployed or without constructive daily activity (Green, Grey, & Wilner, 2002) and seem to reoffend more quickly (Craig & Hutchinson, 2005). They are also less likely to be able to read and write, express themselves verbally, understand abstract or hypothetical concepts, and have problems with memory, learning, problem solving and processing speed. As such, any Circles' projects for people with ID and ASD needs to provide a service that responds to these needs.

In 2012, Circles South East undertook a significant piece of work in order to ascertain whether there was a need to develop a specialist CoSA for these specific client groups, and if so, to consider how such a service may need to differ from its existing model of service delivery. An analysis of all successful referrals to Circles South East was undertaken. Of these 139 individuals, 32 Core Members (approximately 23%) either had a formal diagnosis of ID and/or ASC, or had no formal diagnosis, but evidence existed which strongly suggested the presence of either ID and/or ASC.

Following on from this, Circles South East undertook a further analysis in an attempt to establish whether this population differed in any way in terms of their general characteristics from the non-ID/ASC Core Members. This involved a random selection of ten Core Members with ID/ASC and a comparison group of ten Core Members without ID/ASC. Results of the analysis showed that the individuals with ID and/or ASC displayed a number of general characteristics which set them apart from the non-ID/ASC clients.

These client groups were a significantly younger population, with the average age being 35, compared with an average age of 45 for the comparison group. Despite being younger, the ID/ASC group were more heavily convicted, with 60% having previous convictions for sexual offences, and 40% having previous convictions for other (non-sexual) offences. This compares with 40% having previous convictions for sexual offences, and 30% for non-sexual offences in the comparison group.

Despite being more heavily convicted, those in the ID and/or ASC group were much less likely to be sentenced to a term of imprisonment, with just 30% being sentenced to custody, compared with 80% of the comparison group. They were also much less likely to have completed a recognised sex offending treatment programme either in custody or in the community, with just 50% completing treatment, compared to 90% of the comparison group.

Once Circles South East had been able to establish the prevalence of ID and/or ASC among its Core Members and identify the general characteristics of these individuals, work was undertaken to ascertain whether these clients also experienced different outcomes to their Circles. This piece of work included all 32 of the Core Members initially identified.

When considering outcomes, 56% of the ID/ASC individuals had what could have been considered negative outcomes and behaviours (including recalls to custody, reconvictions, breaches, arrests and disengagement). This was exactly double the amount of negative outcomes and behaviours experienced in the comparison group (28%).

It was also established that of those who successfully completed their Circle, a number went on to commit further offences in the weeks and months following the closure of their Circle. This suggested clear evidence of a need for the development of a model of best practice for Core Members with ID and/or ASC in order to improve successful outcomes.

The Model

In addition to Circles South East, a further five Circles projects have so far offered specialist Circles for people with ID or ASD. These are:

- The Safer Living Foundation (Nottinghamshire and Derbyshire);
- Circles South West;
- North West Circles (CROPT);
- Greater Manchester Circles;
- Respond (London).

What these projects have in common is their approach to working with the Core Member. They also use simplified material including consent forms. A key difference is that these Circles projects take longer: people with ID and ASC need to work at a slower pace, have more support needs and are less likely to be ready to move on after 18 months as on a standard Circle and may need up to two years.

The typical adaptions made by these Circles include simplifying Core Member material so it is accessible such as converting to 'easy-read' format and using simple pictures. Circles South East use a Communication Passport model for all ID/ASC Core Members commencing Circles, which is a collaboratively developed document that outlines all their important support needs and personal information that they can share with the volunteers.

Circles South East have introduced a new Adapted Dynamic Risk Review form to replace the Dynamic Risk Review form (DRR), which is currently used in main Circles. The Adapted DRR is based upon the ARMIDILO-S (Assessment of Risk and Manageability of Intellectually Disabled Individuals who Offend Sexually; Boer, Tough, & Haaven, 2004) a risk assessment tool designed for individuals with learning disabilities.

To date, CoSA have largely been delivered by organisations working in partnership with criminal justice agencies and it is these agencies that provide both funding and referrals. This approach, however, has neglected the needs of men and women with ID/ASC who display harmful sexual behaviour and have not been convicted of a sexual offence, or who have been diverted away from the criminal justice system into health and social care services. The Adapted Circles model could address this problem by providing an additional specialist intervention which aims to meet the needs and reduce the risks of men and women with ID/ASC regardless of their pathway. Circles South East has recently commenced delivery of an Adapted Circles pilot as part of the Hertfordshire Transforming Care Partnership and this is generating referrals for individuals who previously would not have been able to benefit from any form of Circles intervention due to them sitting outside of existing referral pathways. This new approach is enabling a more pro-active approach and engaging with and supporting individuals with ID/ASC prior to criminalisation.

Volunteer Selection and Training

Working with people with ID and ASC can be challenging and volunteers need to demonstrate skills in patience and being able to adapt their style in response to need. Specific training on ID and ASC is essential. This should cover what these disorders are, how they are assessed, and the experiences of people with ID and ASC as well as specific methods for communicating. It is of benefit for volunteers to undertake some skills practice on their training when learning and testing new ways for communicating. For example, having prospective volunteers have a go at using drawing or roleplaying. This builds confidence and comfort with new and sometimes challenging ways of communicating.

Many Core Members with ID/ASC struggle in group settings and can become overwhelmed when introduced to groups of volunteers. In response to this, Circles South East have a gradual introduction of volunteers who are introduced one at a time over a period, which has proved helpful in reducing levels of anxiety. In addition to this, they employ smaller number of volunteers in some Circles as an additional way of reducing anxiety and difficulties coping.

Due to a higher level of impulsivity and disengagement from ID/ASC Core Members, a much greater involvement from Circle Co-ordinators is required and the need to compromise and have a flexible approach in order to keep individuals engaged is paramount.

Outcomes

Formal outcomes have been measured by the SLF and Circles South East. The SLF project has been evaluated by Kitson-Boyce and is commented on it detail in Chap. 4 of this book.

Circles South East are currently running a 3½ year pilot project across Hampshire and Thames Valley. The aim of the pilot was to develop a model of best practice and deliver six 'Adapted Circles' with accompanying evaluation. The Adapted Circles pilot has not yet run to its full conclusion and the evaluation is therefore not currently available.

Transgender Core Members

Client Specific Considerations

The term transgender covers a multitude of gender identifiers and therefore the individual needs are vast for this group. Transgender people who commit offences are an under researched group whose specific forensic needs are unclear. Research in the UK indicates that transgender people are overrepresented in prison in comparison with the community (Poole, Stephens, & Whittle, 2002). Brookes and Jones (2013) found that transgender prisoners have concerns relating to mental health, alcohol and substance abuse problems, are more likely to suffer physical victimisation and stigmatisation and overall have lower life chances. Transgender individuals can be socially ostracised owing to their appearance, lifestyle, or transitional status (Poole et al., 2002). Some transgender individuals do not begin their gender transition until they reach prison. Therefore release may be their first time in the community in their chosen gender(s), which can cause problems reintegrating back into society. Additionally, they may be still transitioning and therefore feel vulnerable and need support. Gender dysphoria is a recognised medical disorder and therefore support is important and required for their continuous transition both physically and mentally.

General resettlement challenges for prisoners can be more difficult for transgender individuals in the community especially in relation to accessing jobs and housing, which may require them to disclose their gender, uncomfortable for some individuals. Housing can cause concerns as these individuals may not get a guaranteed level of privacy (Poole et al., 2002).

Gender dysphoria patients can display personality traits that reflect problems with sense of self. These traits can cause additional support concerns for these individuals as certain problematic behaviours and emotions may be difficult to support and understand. The social difficulties associated with being transgender are thus amplified when they are released from prison, especially if they have committed a sexual offence.

The reasons why some of the transgender population commit sexual offences has not been fully researched to date. This is a difficult area, as some of these individuals would have offended feeling a different gender to how they feel when they are in prison and how they wish to lead the rest of their lives in the community. Specific assessment and consideration needs to be given to each client to consider what rehabilitation pathway would best address their needs, whether this is understood through male sex offending research or female sex offending research.

Due to these complexities, the right level of treatment and rehabilitation may be more difficult to achieve with the usual standardised offending behaviour programmes.

The Model

CoSA could play an important role in supporting transgender people with sexual convictions in the community. These individuals often do not have family and friends to support them in the community. Support is important for this population not only in relation to returning to the community after prison but also in relation to their gender(s). If an individual is transitioning or going into the community for the first time in their chosen gender(s), this is likely to be daunting, as they live and behave in accordance with a new identity, and they may fear the response from the public. The Circle volunteers can provide a positive model of society; someone accepting them as their chosen identity. They might need simple support such as accompanying them to amenities so that they feel confident about being in public and helping them access gender based items such as clothing, make up, and hair styling. They may also need support locating and attending transgender support groups, helping them to make positive connections with the LGBTQ community who will have more knowledge and links with positive transgender specific support.

Volunteer Selection and Training

Coordinator and volunteer understanding and empathy of gender dysphoria will be important as well as their knowledge about supporting those that have offended sexually. Additionally there may be a requirement to have some understanding about the personality traits that clients may present with, as this could impact on their ability to relate to others and use support. However, generally this client group will have similar sexual offending management issues and this will be the main focus in relation to a Circle supporting them. It may be beneficial if a volunteer within their Circle identifies as transgender although this is not a necessity.

It is important for Circles volunteers to have positive attitudes towards working with transgender individuals. A lack of understanding about transgender individuals can lead to negative attitudes which would present as a barrier to the volunteer and client working well together and ensuring positive support is offered. Positive attitudes will also be important as there could be shared stigmatisation and victimisation of the volunteer through their association with this client group. This is something that volunteers need to be aware of before committing to working with this client group. Furthermore, due to the possible social isolation of transgender individuals in the community, it may be that they become dependent on the Circle as their only support, which could cause boundary issues for volunteers. Therefore, a core focus of the Circle should be helping the Core Member to develop support and relationships independent of the Circle.

The Deaf Population[1]

Client Specific Considerations

In Britain, deafness is the second most common disability in the UK with 1 in 1500 people being profoundly, pre-lingually deaf. In 2005, there were 138 prisoners who are d/Deaf compared to 80,000 hearing prisoners. This would suggest an over-representation of people who are deaf in the prison population (Gahir, O'Rourke, Monteiro, & Reed, 2011). Once in prison, it is much more difficult for deaf prisoners to be released (Baines, Patterson, & Austen, 2010). There is some evidence to suggest that social factors, such as a lack of appropriate community support, rehabilitation services, and provision, may have a negative impact on length of incarceration. Research has suggested that an increase in community-based services and provision may well shorten the length of incarceration for deaf clients in the future.

Deaf people tend to have additional support needs related to the psychological, biological and social consequences of being d/Deaf, such as mental health impairment, substance misuse, social isolation, history of physical and sexual abuse, and an inability to read English. They also find accessing resources and services difficult because of the communication barrier therefore they are much less likely to be able to get help for their problems. These factors, coupled with the already disadvantaged social position that having a sexual conviction brings, means that d/Deaf people with sexual convictions are very likely to benefit from the support a Circle could offer but are unlikely to be offered this opportunity.

The Model

It is essential that qualified British Sign Language (BSL) interpreters are used for all interactions and meetings with their Core Member. It is not appropriate to use family or friends as informal interpreters (BPS, 2008). Even if the Core Member has limited BSL skills, an interpreter should still be sought as they can use a variety of methods to aid communication. Core members who have a hearing aid/cochlear implant that enhances residual hearing sufficiently that that they consider English to be their first language, and they do not sign at all, would not need an interpreter. This decision should be led by the Core Member as those who speak English may still benefit from interpreters as they may use Sign Supported English (SSE).

Working with interpreters can bring difficulties, through the addition of a third person in the interpersonal dynamics. The Deaf world is small, but the interpreter world is smaller. There are only around 800 qualified[2] BSL interpreters nationally (Murray, 2013). This means that the d/Deaf client and the interpreter may have met elsewhere, such as socially or in court or may know friends or family members. This can impact on the client's ability to trust the interpreter as they have concerns about whether the interpreter will maintain confidentiality when working elsewhere in the deaf world (Marshall, Fernandez, Hudson, & Ward, 1998). The presence of a third party changes the interpersonal dynamics in ways that hearing people may not be aware. Gold-Brunson and Lawrence (2002) found that despondent interpreter mood caused significant negative mood changes in Deaf clients even when the therapist was cheerful or neutral. Harvey (1982, 1989) also reported on how interpreters may become the object of transference reactions in clients and countertransference reactions in clinicians.

Volunteer Selection

The question of using hearing or d/Deaf volunteers is an important one. The Deaf world is small and groups of Deaf people will travel to other cities to meet other Deaf people at Deaf clubs. Therefore d/Deaf Core Members are more likely to have met, or know by association, any volunteers who are d/Deaf. Rather than being an advantage this can lead to mistrust due to concerns that the volunteer will tell others in the d/Deaf community about their offending. However, it is preferable to use at least one d/Deaf volunteer where possible in a Circle. Rather than being seen as helpers, hearing people have often been involved in oppressing d/Deaf people (Glickman, 2013). Therefore it is likely that having a Deaf volunteer would help break down those barriers between d/Deaf and hearing people. Having someone from the same cultural background would help service users feel more confident that their needs are understood and that there is an awareness of the cultural differences between those in the Circle. There would also be advantages to being able to communicate directly with at least one person in the Circle in terms of building rapport.

Any volunteers would need to demonstrate the same skills as those for standard Circles such as warmth and empathy but in addition, they must be committed to spend time rapport building to develop empathic, respectful, cross-cultural working relationships. Given that hearing people have historically been seen as oppressors, it is important to understand the impact of the special problems d/Deaf people experience to try and reduce this in interactions.

Volunteer Training

In order for the Circles model to be applied with Core Members who are d/Deaf, volunteers require specific training. Deaf awareness training is essential when working with d/Deaf individuals. This aims to improve communication skills and confidence, to help break down the barriers faced daily by people who are d/Deaf or have a hearing loss. The training should cover:

- Terminology: which words are acceptable, which are not;
- Understanding 'Deafness';
- British Sign Language (BSL);
- Communication—tips, strategies and using technology effectively;
- Interpreters and how to work with them.

Communication training is essential as inexperienced people working with d/Deaf individuals often encourage them to lip read and use their voice to avoid the trouble and expense of getting an interpreter. Deaf individuals are vulnerable to acquiescence, compliance and suggestibility (O'Rourke, 2014). If the d/Deaf person acquiesces then the professional may be unaware that good communication is not taking place. The deaf person is merely 'making do' and missing much of the conversation (Critchfield, 2006). In addition to this they are being asked to communicate in their second language, for example English, which they have never heard. This often results in mistaken assumptions such as considering them Intellectually Disabled (ID) (Brennan, Brown, & MacKay, 1997). These issues reduce when interpreters are involved but are unlikely to be removed in their entirety, particularly if questions asked are not d/Deaf friendly. It would also be advantageous for volunteers to learn some basic BSL. This would help build rapport and help address some of the difficulties associated with communicating through a third person.

Conclusions

It is hoped that this chapter has not only provided food for thought for the future of Circles, with new and informative ways of running CoSA, but also practical advice for how to run CoSA for specific minority groups. Providing equal and fair opportunities for those who may have specific requirements or needs is an ongoing issue, not just within the criminal justice system, and it is important that we continue to talk about this. This chapter aimed to shed light on the specific needs some minority groups may have, in order to inform best practice for CoSA.

Notes

1. Those with significant hearing loss often prefer the description 'deaf' or 'Deaf', not 'hearing impaired'. Impaired implies a defect in comparison to hearing people, suggesting that they are an incomplete hearing person. Instead many deaf people see themselves as part of a complete and separate culture and language with a different life experience. For this reason 'deaf' is distinct to 'Deaf' with the latter denoting cultural affiliation.
2. Interpreters should be qualified to level six BSL and have the additional interpreter training. Ensure they are registered with the National Registers

of Communication Professionals working with Deaf and Deafblind People *(NRCPD)*. NRCPD registered BSL/English Interpreters have achieved recognised qualifications and work to strict professional codes of practice. Registration is the only guarantee that providers of communication services have met safe-to-practice standards, have Public Indemnity Insurance and have been subject to Enhanced Criminal Records Bureau (CRB) checks.

References

Almond, L., Canter, D., & Salfati, G. (2006). Youths who sexually harm: A multivariate model of perpetrator characteristics. *Journal of Sexual Aggression, 12*, 97–114.

Baines, D., Patterson, N., & Austen, S. (2010). An investigation into the length of hospital stay for deaf mental health service users. *Journal of Deaf Studies and Deaf Education, 15*(2), 179–184.

Beier, K. M., Neutze, J., Mundt, I. A., Ahlers, C. J., Goecker, D., Konrad, A., et al. (2009). Encouraging self-identified paedophiles and hebephiles to seek professional help: First results of the Prevention Project Dunkelfeld (PPD). *Child Abuse & Neglect, 33*(8), 545–549.

Blake, E., & Gannon, T. A. (2011). Loneliness in sexual offenders. In S. J. Bevinn (Ed.), *Psychology of loneliness* (pp. 49–68). Hauppauge, NY: Nova Science.

Boer, D. P., Tough, S., & Haaven, J. (2004). Assessment of risk manageability of intellectually disabled sexual offenders. *Journal of Applied Research in Intellectual Disabilities, 17*, 275–283.

Brennan, M., Brown, R., & MacKay, B. (1997). *Equality before the law: Deaf people's access to justice*. Durham, UK: Deaf Studies Research Unit.

Brookes, M., & Jones, L. (2013). Transgender offenders: A literature review. *Prison Service Journal, 206*, 11–18.

Cantor, J. (2014). Gold star pedophiles in general sex therapy practice. In Y. Binik & K. Hall (Eds.), *Principles and practice of sex therapy* (5th ed., pp. 219–234). New York: Guilford.

Cantor, J. M., & McPhail, I. V. (2016). Non-offending pedophiles. *Current Sexual Health Reports, 8*(3), 121–128.

Craig, L. A., & Hutchinson, R. (2005). Sexual offenders with learning disabilities: Risk, recidivism and treatment. *Journal of Sexual Aggression, 11*(3), 289–304.

Crawford, T. A. M., & Evans, K. (2016). Crime prevention and community safety. In A. Leibling, S. Maruna, & L. McAra (Eds.), *Oxford handbook of criminology* (6th ed.). Oxford: Oxford University Press. (in press).

Critchfield, A. B. (2006). *Revisiting the dream: Proposing a comprehensive treatment model for deaf, deaf/blind and hard of hearing people who have psychiatric disorders, mental retardation and substance abuse disorders*. Jefferson City: Office of Services to Deaf and Hard of Hearing People, Missouri Department of Mental Health.

Department for Children, School and Families. (2009). Think Family toolkit: Improving support for families at risk examination of adaptive behavior differences in adults with autism spectrum disorders and intellectual disability. *Research in Developmental Disabilities, 30*(9), 1317–1325.

Farrington, D. P. (2007). Childhood risk factors and risk-focused prevention. In M. Maguire, R. Morgan, & R. Reiner (Eds.), *The Oxford handbook of criminology* (4th ed., pp. 602–640). Oxford: Oxford University Press.

Gahir, M., O'Rourke, S., Monteiro, B., & Reed, R. (2011). The unmet needs of deaf prisoners: A survey of prisons in England and Wales. *International Journal on Mental Health and Deafness, 1*(1), 58–63.

Gill v Secretary of State for Justice. (2010). EWHC 364.

Glibert, P. (2009). *The compassionate mind*. London: Constable.

Glickman, N. S. (2013). *Deaf mental health care*. New York: Routledge.

Gold-Brunson, J., & Lawrence, P. S. (2002). Impact of sign language interpreter and therapist moods on deaf recipient mood. *Professional Psychology—Research and Practice, 33*(6), 576–580. https://doi.org/10.1037//0735-7028.33.6.576

Green, G., Gray, N. S., & Willner, P. (2002). Factors associated with criminal convictions for sexually inappropriate behaviour in men with learning disabilities. *The Journal of Forensic Psychiatry, 13*(3), 578–607.

Guay, J. P., Ouimet, M., & Proulx, J. (2004). On intelligence and crime: A comparison of incarcerated sex offenders and serious non-sexual violent criminals. *International Journal of Law and Psychiatry, 28*, 405–417.

Gudjonsson, G. H., & Clare, I. C. H. (1995). The relationship between confabulation and intellectual ability, memory, interrogative suggestibility and acquiescence. *Personal and Individual Differences, 19*(3), 333–338.

Hackett, S. (2014). *Children and young people with harmful sexual behaviours*. London: Research in Practice.

Hackett, S., Philips, J., Masson, H., & Balfe, M. (2013). Individual, family and abuse characteristics of 700 British child and adolescent sexual abusers. *Child Abuse Review, 22*(4), 232–245.

Harvey, M. A. (1982). The influence and utilization of an interpreter for deaf persons in family therapy. *American Annals of the Deaf, 127*(7), 821–827.

Hatzenbuehler, M. L. (2009). How does sexual minority stigma "get under the skin"? A psychological mediation framework. *Psychol Bull, 135*, 707–730.

Holt-Lunstad, J., Smith, T. B., Baker, M., Harris, T., & Stephenson, D. (2015). Loneliness and social isolation as risk factors for mortality: A meta-analytic review. *Perspectives on Psychological Science, 10*(2), 227–237.

Liao, K. Y., Kashubeck-West, S., Weng, C. Y., & Deitz, C. (2015). Testing a mediation framework for the link between perceived discrimination and psychological distress among sexual minority individuals. *Journal of Counseling Psychology, 62*, 226–241.

Lindsay, W. R., Steele, L., Smith, A. H. W., Quinn, K., & Allan, R. (2006). A community forensic intellectual disability service: Twelve year follow up of referrals, analysis of referral patterns and assessment of harm reduction. *Legal and Criminological Psychology, 11*, 113–130.

Mann, R. E., Hanson, K. R., & Thornton, D. (2010). Assessing risk for sexual recidivism: Some proposals on the nature of psychologically meaningful risk factors. *Sex Abuse, 22*, 191–217.

Marshall, W. L. (2010). The role of attachments, intimacy, and loneliness in the etiology and maintenance of sexual offending. *Sexual and Relationship Therapy, 25*, 73–85.

Marshall, W. L., Fernandez, Y. M., Hudson, S. M., & Ward, T. (1998). *Sourcebook of treatment programs for sexual offenders*. London: Plenum Press.

Maruna, S. (2001). *Making good: How ex-convicts reform and rebuild their lives*. Washington, DC: American Psychological Association.

Matson, J. L., Rivet, T. T., Fodstad, J. C., Dempsey, T., & Boisjoli, J. A. (2009). Examination of adaptive behaviour differences in adults with autism spectrum disorders and intellectual disability. *Research in Developmental Disabilities, 30*(9), 1317–1325.

Maulik, P. K., Mascarenhas, M. N., Mathers, D. D., Dua, T., & Saxena, S. (2011). Prevalence of intellectual disability: A meta-analysis of population-based studies. *Research in Developmental Disabilities, 32*(2), 419–436.

McAra, L., & McVie, S. (2012). Critical debates in developmental and life-course criminology. In M. Maguire, R. Morgan, & R. Reiner (Eds.), *The Oxford handbook of criminology* (5th ed., pp. 531–560). Oxford: Oxford University Press.

McPhail, I. V., Hermann, C. A., Fernane, S., Fernandez, Y. M., Nunes, K. L., & Cantor, J. M. (2017). Validity in phallometric testing for sexual interests in children: A meta-analytic review. *Assessment*. https://doi.org/10.1177/1073191117706139

Mouridsen, S. E. (2012). Current status of research on autism spectrum disorders and offending. *Research in Autism Spectrum Disorders, 6*(1), 79–86.

Murray, K. (2013, May 7). Lack of British Sign Language interpreters putting deaf people at risk. *The Guardian*. Retrieved from http://www.theguardian.com/society/2013/may/07/lack-interpreters-deaf-people-risk

NSPCC. (2011). NSPCC finds 64 child sex crimes a day recorded by police. *NSPCC press release*, 26 May 2011. London: NSPCC.

O'Rourke, S. (2014). *Planning to question someone who is Deaf.* Retrieved March 3, 2016, from http://www.theadvocatesgateway.org/toolkits

Perrin, C., Blagden, N., Winder, B., & Dillon, G. (2017). "It's sort of reaffirmed to me that I'm not a monster, I'm not a terrible person": Sex offenders' movements toward desistance via peer-support roles in prison. *Sexual Abuse.* https://doi.org/10.1177/1079063217697133

Poole, L., Stephens, P., & Whittle, S. (2002). Working with transgendered and transsexual people as offenders in the probation service. *Probation Journal, 49*(3), 227–232.

Rich, P. (2011). *Understanding, assessing and rehabilitating juvenile sexual offenders.* Hoboken, NJ: Wiley.

Righthand, S., & Welch, C. (2001). *Juveniles who have sexually offended: A review of the professional literature.* Washington, DC: Office of Juvenile Justice and Delinquency Prevention.

Seto, M. C. (2008). *Pedophilia and sexual offending against children: Theory, assessment, and intervention.* Washington, DC: American Psychological Association.

Stevens, A. (2012). *Offender rehabilitation and therapeutic communities: Enabling change the TC way.* Oxford: Routledge.

The British Psychological Society. (2008). *Working with interpreters in health settings: Guidelines for psychologists.* Leicester, UK: BPS.

Tracy, K., & Wallace, S. P. (2016). Benefits of peer support groups in the treatment of addiction. *Substance Abuse and Rehabilitation, 7*, 143–154. https://doi.org/10.2147/SAR.S81535

Veneziano, C., & Veneziano, L. (2002). Adolescent sex offenders: A review of literature. *Trauma, Violence and Abuse Journal, 3*, 247–260.

Volkmar, F., & Dykens. (2002). Mental retardation. In M. Rutter & E. Taylor (Eds.), *Child and adolescent psychiatry* (4th ed., pp. (697–(710). Oxford: Blackwell.

Ward, T., Keenan, T., & Hudson, S. M. (2000). Understanding cognitive affective, and intimacy deficits in sexual offenders: A developmental perspective. *Aggression and Violent Behavior, 5*, 41–62. https://doi.org/10.1016/S1359-1789(98)00025-1

Ward, T., & Stewart, C. A. (2003). The treatment of sex offenders: Risk management and good lives. *Professional Psychology, Research and Practice, 34*, 353–360.

Winder, B., Lievesley, R., Elliott, H., Hocken, K., Faulkner, J., Norman, C., et al. (2017). Evaluation of the use of pharmacological treatment with prisoners experiencing high levels of hypersexual disorder. *The Journal of Forensic Psychiatry & Psychology, 29*(1), 53–71. https://doi.org/10.1080/14789949.2017.1337801

Glossary

Agency A sense of agency is a belief that one is capable of exerting influence upon one's self and environment.

The availability heuristic A mental process whereby familiar or more common stimuli are processed more quickly than unfamiliar or less common stimuli.

Availability cascade The process by which a high-profile case leads to a succession of political discussions and legislative changes, typically brought about by lobbying from powerful stakeholders.

The representativeness heuristic A mental process whereby stimuli are intuitively categorised based on their closeness to stereotypes.

The affect heuristic A mental process whereby decisions are made on the basis of automatic positive or negative feelings about a given objector issue.

Community notification laws Legislation that allows or requires the public to have access to information about those who are registered as sexual offenders. The specific enactment of these procedures varies between states.

Criminogenic needs Criminogenic needs are dynamic risk factors that are empirically related to recidivism. These risk factors are amenable to treatment and include deviant sexual interests, distorted attitudes and beliefs, anti-social lifestyle and problems with self-regulation.

Narrative humanisation The process of overcoming dehumanised stereotypes by humanising a target group through the presentation of personal life stories.

H. Elliott et al. (eds.), *Sexual Crime and Circles of Support and Accountability*, Sexual Crime, https://doi.org/10.1007/978-3-319-74823-8

Protective factors Protective factors are social, interpersonal, and environmental factors, as well as psychological and behavioural features that are empirically linked to sexual offending. They differ from risk factors/criminogenic needs in that they are based on positive aspects of the individual and/or existing social capital.

Core Member An individual who has been convicted of a sexual offence receiving support through the Circles of Support and Accountability initiative to successfully reintegrate back into society post-release from prison.

Transference The process whereby a client experiences their therapist as similar to, or exactly like a significant caregiver from their childhood. For example they may experience their therapist as overly critical or withholding.

Countertransference This is where the therapist experiences transference towards their client. This may be based on the therapist's own history (as per the definition of transference), or it may be the therapist reacting to the transference within the client.

Index[1]

A

Acceptance, 16, 33, 54, 58, 62, 84, 86, 90
Accommodation, 12, 16, 93, 106, 157, 159, 166–168
Accountability, 1–21, 30, 35, 48, 51
Accountable, 90, 92, 105–122, 151–169, 179, 181, 182, 189
Activities/activity, 7, 10, 18, 29, 57, 59, 113, 115, 144, 172, 173, 184–186
Adapted Circles, 189, 190
Affiliation, 173
Anxiety, 85, 86, 88, 91, 94, 97, 110, 134, 172, 173, 175, 178, 180, 182, 190
Approved premises, 77, 92
Assertive, 129
Assessment, 18, 19, 44, 45, 50, 76, 78, 107, 108, 140, 189, 191
Assessment of Risk and Manageability of Intellectually Disabled Individuals who Offend Sexually (ARMIDILO-S), 189
Attachment, 10, 74, 172–174, 184
Attitude, 4, 29–31, 36, 56, 57, 63, 84, 107, 127, 128, 133–135, 139–145, 161, 163, 182, 185, 192, 193
Attrition, 117–119
Autistic spectrum conditions (ASC), 185–190

[1] Note: Page number followed by 'n' refer to notes.

H. Elliott et al. (eds.), *Sexual Crime and Circles of Support and Accountability*, Sexual Crime, https://doi.org/10.1007/978-3-319-74823-8

B

Belonging, 26, 30, 31, 33, 34, 55, 56, 58, 92, 119, 174
Benefits, 12, 16, 26, 53, 56, 61, 63, 64, 77, 82, 83, 85, 87–89, 96–98, 112, 116, 122, 134, 140, 167, 173–176, 181, 185, 186, 189, 190, 193, 194
Best practice, 17, 43, 56, 151, 188, 190, 196
Britain/British, 4, 5, 11, 14, 17, 20, 21, 128, 131, 134, 142, 193
British Sign Language (BSL), 194–196
British tabloid, 128
Broadsheet newspaper, 128

C

Canada, 1, 6, 11, 43, 45, 47
  Canadian, 3–5, 7, 9, 13, 17, 20, 21, 47, 51, 73
Child Sex Offender Disclosure Scheme, 131
Circles 4EU, 20
Circles UK, 14, 17–19, 21, 107, 122, 161
Code of practice, 19
Cognitive-Experiential Self-Theory, 129
Communication, 12, 36, 58, 96, 141, 186, 188, 193–196
Community, 2–10, 12, 13, 15, 16, 18, 21, 26–37, 53–55, 59–63, 71–98, 105–122, 130, 131, 137–139, 143–145, 151–169, 172, 174–181, 183–187, 191–193, 195
Confidence, 12, 16, 43, 113, 185, 190, 195
  self-confidence, 59
Contact, 45, 48–50, 60, 74, 78, 82, 110, 114, 158, 163, 173
Control, 2, 10, 13, 35, 47, 48, 52, 53, 64, 108, 113, 114, 142, 164, 175, 178
Control group, 51–53, 64, 108, 142
Coordinator, 18, 19, 26, 33, 61, 79, 82, 122, 151–169, 174, 192
Coping skills, 57, 113, 115
Core Members, 8, 26, 44, 72, 106, 114, 138, 151, 172
Courses, 9, 57, 107, 157, 159, 160, 167, 172
Crime, 8, 9, 15, 25, 26, 28–36, 44, 45, 52–60, 62, 64, 71, 74, 91, 94, 95, 97, 111, 127–137, 139, 141, 143, 145, 156, 160, 172, 176–178, 186
Criminal history, 55
Criminal justice, 2–4, 6, 9, 76, 163, 165, 174, 176, 177, 179, 182, 189
Criminogenic, 2, 10, 13–15, 25, 35, 36
Criticism/critique, 13, 49, 53, 56, 64, 77

D

Deaf, 172, 193–196
Dehumanisation, 135, 136
Dehumanised, 136, 142, 143
Denial, 11, 63, 158
Desistence
  moral agency, 27
  personal agency, 2

Disclosure/disclose, 10, 89, 130, 182, 184, 191
Drop-out, 118
Dual-process cognition, 128–129
Dynamic risk, 13, 107–108, 116, 189
Dynamic Risk Review (DRR), 107, 108, 116, 189

E
Education, 18, 56, 57, 63, 128, 132, 155
Effectiveness, 20, 30, 49–51, 53, 62–64, 93, 96, 97, 106, 108, 116, 122, 140
Efficacy, 43, 45, 47, 49–51, 54, 59, 138, 178
Elaboration Likelihood Model, the, 129
Elderly, 75–78
Emotion, 10, 26, 30, 34, 54–57, 95, 106, 108, 110, 112, 113, 115, 116, 119, 122, 134, 136, 137, 139, 141, 145, 178, 180–183, 185, 191
Employment, 12, 25, 56, 63, 71, 106
Ending, 29, 117, 166
England, 6, 17–19, 75, 76, 116
Equality, 9, 58, 179, 185
Europe, 3, 12, 19, 86
  European, 4, 7, 19, 20
Evaluation
  mixed methods, 106
  outcome evaluation, 106
  process evaluation, 106
Ex-offender, 7, 37, 48, 72, 74, 83, 86, 95, 98, 111–115
External, 25, 28, 58–60, 114

F
Failure, 48, 51, 106, 108, 116, 117, 119, 120
Friendship/friend, 52, 83, 93, 110, 121, 138, 144, 159, 161

G
Gender, 179, 185, 190–192
Gender dysphoria, 191, 192
Good Friday Agreement, 7
Good Lives Model (GLM), 10, 14, 36, 182
  basic needs, 15
Government, 5–8, 15–17, 21, 62, 136
Group, 52

H
Hamilton, 1
Hamilton, Ontario, 4
Harmful sexual behaviour (HSB), 180–182, 189
Healthy, 10, 55
Her Majesty's Prison and Probation Service (HMPPS), 6
Heuristics
  affect heuristics, 134, 141, 142
  availability Heuristic, 129, 131, 137
  representative Heuristics, 128
Heuristic-Systematic Model, 129

High-profile, 1, 17, 130–132, 137, 139
HMP Whatton, 18, 74, 167, 182
Home Office, 5–7, 11, 16, 17
Hope, 57, 58, 161, 166, 169
Housing, 12, 63, 71, 86, 92–94, 97, 144, 156, 191
Human goods, 15, 36, 143
Human rights, 8, 135, 136, 179

I

Identity, 13, 25–29, 31, 37, 58, 72, 74, 90, 95, 111, 115, 118, 174, 192
Implicit cognition, 141
Implicit theories, 133
Imprisonment, 36, 49, 136, 187
Inclusion, 8, 10, 31, 33, 34, 37, 51, 55, 90, 115, 119, 141, 179, 183
Information processing, 128, 129, 139
Innovation Means Prisons and Communities (IMPACT), 7
Insight, 57
Institutionalised, 2, 166
Integrated Theory of Desistance from Sexual Offending (the) (ITDSO), 28
Intellectual disability (ID), 2, 75–78, 81, 88, 89, 185–190, 196
Internal, 25, 58, 59, 113, 114
Interpersonal, 32, 59, 178, 194
Interpretative Phenomenological Analysis (IPA), 81
Interpreter, 194–196
Intervention, 15, 26, 30, 31, 35, 48, 53, 60, 105–107, 116, 117, 119, 142, 178, 182, 183, 189
Interviews, 55, 57–59, 77, 81, 84, 113, 119, 151, 152, 158, 164, 167–169
  semi-structured, 80
Intimacy, 10
IQ, 78, 186
Isolation, 2, 10, 75, 112
  social isolation, 34, 54–56, 63, 71, 76, 82, 94, 96, 113, 173, 181–183, 193

K

Kindness, 173
Kitchener probation office, 3

L

Label/labelling, 26, 29, 33, 37, 95, 110–112, 115, 134–137, 144
Leisure, 57, 59, 186
LGBTQ, 192
Licence, 47
  licence conditions, 51, 88, 96, 168, 181
Locus of Control (LOC), 113, 114
Loneliness, 2, 10, 54–56, 63, 72, 76, 82, 96, 172, 178, 181–183, 185
Lucy Faithfull Foundation, 6

M

Maintain, 9, 10, 16, 18, 28, 72, 143, 172, 194
Management of Sexual Offenders and Violent Offenders (MOSOVO), 35, 168
Maslow's hierarchy of needs, 111

Media, 5, 18, 19, 30, 55, 62, 71, 85, 94, 111, 112, 127–145
Media campaign, 1, 5, 131, 177
Mediation, 1, 3, 4, 9
Medication to manage sexual arousal, 178
Medium risk, 79
Megan's Law, 131
Memory, 159, 186
  recall, 129
Mennonite, 3, 4, 21
Mental health, 112–114, 185, 191, 193
Mental systems, 129
Mentoring, 29, 72, 175
Ministry of Justice, 17, 57
Modelling, 10, 72
Monitor, 9–12, 107
Motivation, 29, 45, 50–55, 57, 58, 60, 72, 91, 117, 176
Multi Agency Public Protection Arrangements (MAPPA), 5, 10, 11, 13, 15, 17, 19, 20, 35, 163

N

Narrative, narrative identity, 25–27
National Offender Management service (NOMS), 6
National Probation Service, 19, 108
Neurodevelopmental, 185
Non-contact, 45, 50
Non-offending, 16, 142, 174, 177
Not-In-My-Backyard' (NIMBYism), 137–139
Nottingham Trent University, 75, 77, 78
NSPCC, 180

O

Offender identity, 95, 118, 174
Offender Managers, 108
Openness, 57–59, 96

P

Paedophile, 5, 33, 137, 138, 142
Paedophilia, 142, 177
Paedophilic, 141, 174
Parliament, 16, 17
Parole, 47, 48, 165, 166
Personality, 132, 133, 174, 191, 192
Police, 6, 12, 17–19, 50, 75, 87, 88, 131, 157, 159
Prejudice, 111, 112
Prevention Project Dunkelfeld, 176, 177
Prison, 2, 4, 5, 7, 11, 12, 16, 28, 32, 48, 50–52, 55, 57, 61, 72–94, 96–98, 107, 108, 110, 115, 117, 136, 137, 154–156, 158, 160, 161, 164–167, 174, 179, 191–193
Prison-based CoSA, 73, 76, 82
Prison Reform Trust, 76
Probation, 3, 6, 7, 11–13, 15, 17–20, 29, 75, 85–87, 117, 159, 161, 163, 168
Probation officer, 3, 85–87, 159, 161, 163
Problem solving, 57, 59, 115, 119, 186
Process, 8–10, 13, 17, 19, 20, 25–32, 34, 35, 44, 52, 53, 58, 72, 77, 79, 86, 89, 93, 106, 108, 113, 118, 127–129, 132–135, 137, 139, 140, 143, 145, 175, 184, 186

Professionals, 2, 3, 5, 16, 60, 83, 106, 112, 119–122, 132, 144, 161, 196, 197n2
Pro-social, 26, 28, 31, 34, 36, 55, 56, 58, 74, 82–84, 90, 91, 96, 98, 111, 120, 182
Protective factors, 26, 34, 115, 118, 183
Psychologically informed Circles, 172–174
Psychologically Informed Planned Environments (PIPES), 174
Psychological processes, 127, 128
Public attitudes, 140, 141, 145
Public perception, 4, 62, 63, 130, 169
Public protection, 10, 13

Q

Quakers, 5–7, 17, 18, 77, 163
Qualitative, 27, 43, 45, 54–56, 58, 64, 77
Quantitative, 54, 56, 58–60, 64, 77
Questionnaire, 58, 60

R

Randomised Control Trail (RCT), 51–54, 73
Rapport, 84–87, 195, 196
Reactive, 10, 176
Recidivism, 13, 31, 35, 43–49, 52, 54, 56, 77, 78, 83, 106, 108, 113, 114, 116, 118, 120–122, 144
Recidivist, 1, 10, 47, 54, 55, 182
Reconviction, 47–50, 52, 75, 95, 97, 108, 188
Recruitment, 118, 139, 144, 145, 177, 184
Redemptive, 27
Re-entering, 84, 91, 92
Re-entry, 28, 35–36, 72, 83, 95, 97, 143
Rehabilitation/rehabilitative, 9, 10, 13–16, 21, 25, 26, 28–32, 35–37, 46, 63, 86, 97, 108, 119, 136–138, 140, 143, 145, 174–176, 182, 191–193
Reintegration/reintegrated, 3, 8, 10, 15, 16, 25–27, 32–34, 48, 54, 55, 59–63, 71, 73, 76, 83, 92–98, 115, 118, 120, 137–140, 144, 168, 169, 173, 191
Relapse prevention, 14, 57
Relapse prevention plan, 14, 57
Relationship/relational, 8, 10, 32, 55, 57
Release, 44, 51, 73, 87
Reoffending, 2, 10, 15, 28, 32, 33, 36, 44, 52, 55, 60, 97, 106, 144, 167
Re-settling, 90
Restoration, 48
Restorative, retributive justice, 9
Reverend Harry Nigh, 1, 3, 4
Risk assessment, 19, 76, 78, 107, 140, 189
Risk factors, 15, 34, 54, 82, 107, 113, 172, 178
Risk management, 2, 5, 9, 12, 16, 20, 48, 92, 120
Risk, Needs and Responsivity (RNR), 10, 13
RM2000, 50, 76, 78, 79

S

Safer Living Foundation, the (SLF), 18, 75, 151–169, 188
"Sarah's Law", 131
Scotland, 7, 116
Self-change, 26, 32, 33
Self-determination, 30
Self-esteem, 12, 60, 85, 86, 106, 110, 113, 119, 175, 185
Self-identity, 26
Sentence
  prison sentence, 44, 76, 85, 136
  sentencing, 13, 133, 137, 153
Sex offender prevention orders (SOPO), 10
Sex Offender Treatment Programme (SOTP), 6, 13, 15, 28, 44, 45, 58, 89, 97, 155, 156, 159, 160, 167
Sexual abuse, 4, 5, 48, 49, 168, 177, 178, 180, 193
Sexual crime, 29, 30, 32, 33, 36, 44, 45, 52, 53, 60, 62, 71, 111, 127–137, 139, 141, 143, 172, 176, 177
Sexual offence, 2, 4, 5, 7, 13, 20, 26–28, 30, 44, 46, 47, 49–56, 61–63, 71–78, 82, 84–86, 88, 91, 92, 94, 95, 97, 98, 106, 107, 110, 111, 113–115, 117, 121, 127–129, 131, 133–143, 145, 164, 169, 174–176, 178, 181, 182, 186, 187, 189, 191
Sexual offender, 28, 29, 127, 133, 134, 141, 144, 164
Shame, 5, 32, 33, 172, 177, 178
  disintegrative shaming, 33
Social bonds, 56, 58, 74, 79, 91, 96
Social capital, 15, 34, 37, 60, 71
Social isolation, 34, 54–56, 63, 71, 76, 82, 94, 96, 113, 173, 180, 182, 183, 193
Social network, 31, 34, 59, 72, 75, 106
Social skills, 59, 113, 119, 180, 182
Society, 15, 26, 29, 33, 34, 55, 59, 61, 71, 73, 83, 90, 92, 94, 96, 97, 110, 111, 130, 143, 168, 169, 180, 181, 191, 192
Stakeholder, 2, 3, 8, 9, 105, 120, 130
STATIC-99, 45
Static risk, 76, 78, 107
Statutory, 2, 5, 6, 9, 11, 13, 92
Stereotype, 85, 127, 132, 133, 136, 139, 143
Stereotypical, 127, 133, 134
Stigma/stigmatisation, 28, 29, 32, 33, 61–63, 71, 85, 88, 92, 94–97, 110–112, 120, 121, 142, 177, 178, 191, 193
Stimuli, 129, 132, 141
Strength-based, 13, 15, 35
Strength-based approach, 15, 36, 118, 121, 182
Stress, 57, 59, 61, 118, 162, 166
Structured Assessment of Risk and Need (SARN), 107
Success, 3, 6–8, 11–17, 19, 20, 25, 26, 28, 29, 31, 32, 43, 45, 47–49, 54–60, 63, 64, 71–75, 83, 84, 90, 92–98, 105, 106, 108, 116–117, 119, 120, 122, 130, 137, 140, 144, 145, 168, 173, 175–177, 181, 184, 187, 188
Supervision, 4, 11, 35, 61, 62, 92, 174

Survive, 59, 172
System 1/System 2 Theory, 129

T

Taylor, Charlie, 1, 2
  Charlie's Angels, 1
Thames Valley, 6, 7, 11, 13, 16, 18, 47, 190
Thematic analysis, 55
Therapeutic alliance, 13, 14, 30
Therapeutic environment, 118
Through the Gate, 11, 18, 73
Together in Safety, 19
Training, 12, 14, 17–20, 89, 120, 121, 152, 164, 167, 168, 172, 179, 182, 184–185, 189, 190, 192–193, 195–196, 196n2
Transformation, 8–10, 13, 14, 25, 27
Transgender, 191–193
Transition, 8, 25–37, 58, 59, 71–98, 119, 138, 156, 191, 192
Treatment, 4, 6, 10, 11, 14, 15, 30, 35, 44, 45, 47, 53, 58, 72, 74, 78, 86, 96, 97, 115, 117–119, 136–138, 141, 175–179, 186, 187, 192
Trust, 8, 17, 32, 34, 58, 73, 86, 94, 119, 159, 163, 172, 173, 194
Turning point, 27

U

United Kingdom (UK), 5, 6, 13, 108

V

Validation, 32
Values, 5, 7–10, 14, 20
Victim, 3–5, 8, 9, 21, 44, 48, 50, 57, 60, 62, 63, 83, 114, 135, 145, 154, 158, 168, 169, 175, 176, 178, 182
Victimisation, 63, 191, 193
Victim/Offender Reconciliation Project (VORP), 3, 4
Victim Services Programme, 4
Violent and Sexual Offenders Register (ViSOR), 136
Virped, 177
Volunteer, 1–4, 7, 8, 10–16, 18, 26, 28–33, 36, 48, 53, 55–64, 73, 74, 77, 79, 83–87, 89–93, 96, 97, 106, 112–114, 116–119
Volunteer training, 89, 195–196
Vulnerabilities, 173, 178
Vulnerable, 64, 75, 86, 116, 139, 169, 180, 191, 196

W

Wales, 17, 19, 75, 76, 78, 137
Warwick-Edinburgh Mental Well-Being Scale (WEMWBS), 115, 116
Wellbeing
  eudaimonic, 112, 113
  hedonic, 112
We-ness, 31, 83
What Works, 15, 35, 152, 177
Withdraw, 58, 118
Withdrawal, 50, 117

Y

Young people, 172, 180–184, 186
Young People's Circles, 181–185

The manufacturer's authorised representative in the EU is Springer Nature Customer Service Centre GmbH, Europaplatz 3, 69115 Heidelberg, Germany. If you have any concerns regarding our products, please contact ProductSafety@springernature.com

Printed and bound by CPI Group (UK) Ltd, Croydon, CR0 4YY
30/09/2026
02225660-0005